Prepared by Jane M. Hemminger, RD, LD

FOOD SAFETY: A GUIDE TO WHAT YOU REALLY NEED TO KNOW

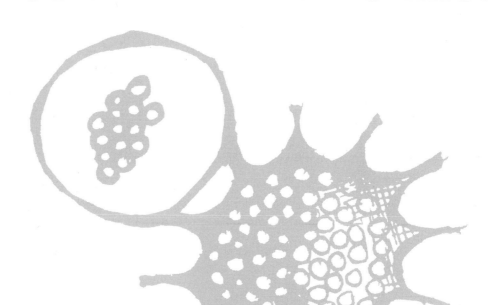

Approved by the Iowa Dietetic Association

Reviewed for Publication by:

Bonnie Moeller, RD, LD
Anne Shaner, RD, LD
Betty Barton
Judy Walrod, RD, LD
Jill Gabel, RD, LD
Pat Moreland, MPA, RD, LD

Iowa State University Press, Ames

Jane M. Hemminger is a graduate of Iowa State University with a degree in food and nutrition. She received her sanitation certification from the state of Illinois. Hemminger is a foods consultant working on food, nutrition, and sanitation projects. She is an experienced supervisor of sanitation programs and has conducted sanitation inservices.

© 2000 Iowa State University Press

Iowa State University Press
2121 South State Avenue, Ames, Iowa 50014

Orders: 1-800-862-6657
Office: 1-515-292-0140
Fax: 1-515-292-3348
Web site: www.isupress.edu

Authorization to photocopy items for internal or personal use, or the internal or personal use of specific clients, is granted by Iowa State University Press, provided that the base fee of $.10 per copy is paid directly to the Copyright Clearance Center, 222 Rosewood Drive, Danvers, MA 01923. For those organizations that have been granted a photocopy license by CCC, a separate system of payments has been arranged. The fee code for users of the Transactional Reporting Service is 0-8138-2482-6/99 $.10.

♾ Printed on acid-free paper in the United States of America

First edition, 2000

Library of Congress Cataloging-in-Publication Data
Hemminger, Jane M.
    Food safety: a guide to what you really need to know / prepared by Jane M. Hemminger; approved by the Iowa Dietetic Association; reviewed for publication by Bonnie Moeller— [et al.].—1st ed.
        p. cm.
    ISBN 0-8138-2482-6
    1. Food service—Safety measures—Handbooks, manuals, etc. 2. Food service—Sanitation—Handbooks, manuals, etc. I. Title.
    TX911.3.S24 H46 1999
    647.95'068'4—dc21
                                                                99-045971

The last digit is the print number: 9 8 7 6 5 4 3 2 1

FOOD SAFETY: A GUIDE TO WHAT YOU REALLY NEED TO KNOW

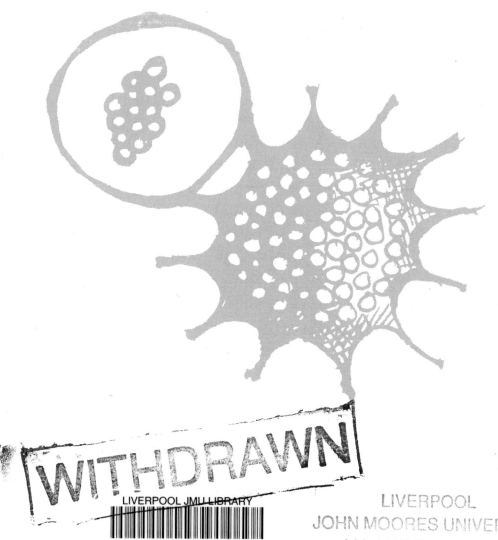

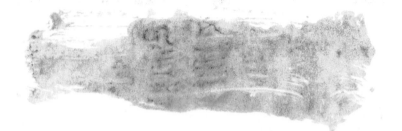

Contents

Acknowledgments   vii

Introduction   ix

1 Food Hazards   3

2 Foodborne Illnesses   11

3 Preparation and Service of Safe Food   21

4 Cleaning and Sanitation   39

5 Safety   51

6 Facilities and Equipment   55

7 Trash Removal   59

8 Pest Control   63

9 Inspections   67

Appendix 1—Hazard Analysis Critical Control Points Flowchart   71

Appendix 2—Sanitation Walk-Through   73

Appendix 3—Maximum Recommended Storage Times (Refrigerator/Freezer)   85

Appendix 4—Maximum Recommended Storage Times (Storeroom)   86

Study Question Answers   87

Glossary   89

References   95

Acknowledgments

Thank you to Linda Setchell for her knowledge, assistance, and friendship—all are of great value.

Thanks to Pam Carberry, Phillip Chase, and Calvin Community retirement center for proofreading, suggestions, and providing kitchen workspace for hands-on use.

Thanks to John Van Cleave for his artwork. John is a graduate of Roosevelt High School in Des Moines, Iowa, and is attending Minneapolis College of Art.

Thank you to Michael Leaders of Hawkeye Foods and Jeff Fleming from Ecolab, Inc., for their willingness to pass along helpful information. It was much appreciated.

My appreciation to Jim Ice at ISU Press for his insight and helpfulness along the way.

Thank you to Bonnie Moeller and the Iowa Dietetic Association for the opportunity to work on this project.

I would also like to thank Bonnie Moeller, Anne Shaner, Betty Barton, Judy Walrod, Jill Gabel, and Pat Moreland for their time and expertise in reviewing this manual.

Let's play 13 questions! (That 20 questions thing has been so overdone.)

Question #1:
What is the significance of the range 5.6–9.4 billion?

A. It is the number of questions you are asked per day.
 Close.

B. It is the number of employees you go through until you find a good one.
 Maybe.

C. It is the average salary of a foodservice supervisor.
 Nope!

It is none of the above. It is, however, the number of dollars spent each year on the major foodborne illnesses. According to the Economic Research Service of the United States Department of Agriculture (USDA) 5.6–9.4 billion dollars a year are spent on medical costs and lost productivity costs associated with the top seven foodborne illnesses. That is an amazing amount of money to waste on bad practices.

These costs don't include the financial ripple effect of media exposure. A single evening news story or an article in the local paper about an incident of foodborne illness can have a devastating effect on business for months. People forget these incidents over time, but not before they have taken their business, and possibly their loyalty, elsewhere. Not many foodservice operations can handle a prolonged boycott.

It isn't all about money either. It is, more importantly, about people—people getting sick needlessly. And in some populations, especially the elderly, young children, and already compromised individuals, it can be life threatening. That is something for which no one wants to claim responsibility.

Even though we work in the food industry, we are also customers to it. Just like anyone, we are exposed, at one time or another, to the food handling techniques of someone else. From those experiences, good or bad, we can learn how to become better food handlers ourselves.

The purpose of this manual is to help foodservice managers put appropriate techniques into practice and serve safe food while at the same time creating a safe work environment for employees and the products they produce.

Question #2:
What, then, is the significance of 500–900 billion?

A. It is the number of ways to serve leftover Thanksgiving turkey.
 Fortunately not.

B. It is the average salary of foodservice supervisors after they learn the material in this manual.
 Doubt it.

C. It is the number of safe meals served yearly by knowledgeable foodservice personnel.
 Hopefully.

FOOD SAFETY: A GUIDE TO WHAT YOU REALLY NEED TO KNOW

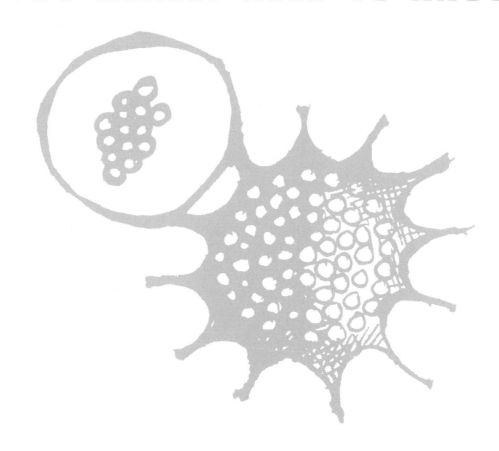

Chapter One:
Food Hazards

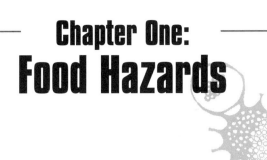

anything that interferes with food safety is a food hazard

LEARNING OBJECTIVES

After this chapter you should be able to

- Identify the three types of food hazards,
- Identify ways to prevent food hazards from harming the food supply,
- Know the difference between food infection and intoxication,
- Understand the elements needed for bacterial growth, and
- Describe potentially hazardous foods.

If we were to modify that famous line from *A Field of Dreams* for foodservice use, it might say, "If you cook it, they will come." But a second line would surely follow, "If you make them sick, they will leave." Foodborne illnesses are a manager's worst nightmare. Unfortunately, however, until they've experienced that nightmare, many people assign a low priority to food safety. Working through the causes of food safety problems and using appropriate techniques to prevent them is the only way to ensure safe food. Anything that interferes with the service of safe foods is a **food hazard**. These hazards are divided into three categories:

- Physical hazards,
- Chemical hazards, and
- Biological hazards.

Any one of these hazards can be involved in a food safety problem.

PHYSICAL HAZARDS

Anything foreign to the food can be considered a physical hazard. Dust, dirt, hair, metal shavings, and broken glass, for example, are items foreign to the original food and are considered harmful. Contamination with such accidental items can almost always be avoided by using good techniques such as those shown below.

Dust
Keep the work areas clean. Wipe shelving, racks, cupboards, and especially exhaust and heating/cooling vents. Wipe the tops of cans before opening.

Dirt
Keep things clean. Wash counters, carts, and cabinets frequently. Clean fresh produce thoroughly before using. Wash hands frequently.

Hair

Keep it restrained. It is the item we least like to find in our food, but it is the hardest to get people to do anything about. All hair needs to be kept restrained in a manner that is compatible with local health codes (using hairnets, caps, etc.).

Metal shavings

Clean can openers daily and change blades as they become dull. If the facility recycles, keep empty cans and can-crushing equipment away from preparation areas.

Broken glass

Use as many unbreakable containers as possible. Use only plastic or metal scoops when dipping into an ice bin. Discard broken, chipped, or cracked items (dinnerware, glassware, serving dishes, etc.). Maintain a separate LABELED receptacle for broken glass.

Foreign objects

Everyone has heard a funny story of someone finding something weird in their food. It is, however, only amusing if the story is not about you or your facility. So keep foreign materials (twist ties, toothpicks, box staples, bottle rings, stones, etc.) away from preparation areas. Handle these items once, discarding or using them immediately. Rinse and pick through dried beans, checking carefully for stones.

Hygiene

Limit jewelry to a minimum—only post earrings and other non-dangling jewelry (dangling jewelry can get caught in equipment). Keep fingernails trimmed, clean and unpolished; no false fingernails should be worn in any area of the foodservice operation. Keep cuts and bandages covered with a disposable glove and change gloves frequently.

CHEMICAL HAZARDS

Chemical hazards are just what the name implies—a food hazard that is the result of exposure to or absorption of chemicals. What probably comes to mind most often are cleaning solutions, but chemical hazards also include pesticides, toxic metals, and some food additives. The techniques listed below will help avoid chemical hazards.

Cleaning solutions

Always keep cleaning solutions stored separately from food products both in the storeroom and in the work area. Do not transfer cleaning solutions out of their original containers unless they are being put into a clear LABELED container that is not to be reused in food preparation. All cleaning solutions must be kept away from the preparation of food. Anyone using cleaning compounds must wash and dry their hands before handling food.

Pesticides

As much as possible, pest control should be handled at times when food preparation is not being done. All foods must be covered before pesticide application, and all food contact surfaces must be washed and sanitized before food preparation can restart.

Pesticides can also come to us on fresh fruits and vegetables. Purchase produce from reputable suppliers and THOROUGHLY wash before preparation—this includes washing the outsides of items that will be peeled (melons, for example) since the contaminant can be carried from the outer peel to the fruit on the knife blade.

Toxic metals

There are many metals that can be nutritionally beneficial in very small amounts; these same metals in large concentrations can prove to be harmful. The most commonly involved metals are

- Zinc — Zinc is found in galvanized containers (pots, pans, etc.). When these containers come in contact with high-acid foods, they can produce harmful zinc salts. Never put high-acid foods (lemonade, tomatoes, fruit juices, chicken, etc.) into galvanized containers.
- Cadmium — Cadmium is found in rust-proof items such as ice cube trays and pitchers. It can cause poisoning when fumes are inhaled. Do not use these products in commercial operations.
- Lead — Lead can be found in pewter or lead-glazed china. Never use these items for cooking or serving food.
- Mercury — The presence of mercury, which was a serious problem years ago, is often a result of water pollution and requires the use of reputable seafood suppliers.

Food additives

Food additives are present in many foods to alter, enhance, or preserve the taste of the item. Other additives are a part of a food product by accident—coming as residuals from pesticides, herbicides, and drugs given to livestock. These "accidental additives" can be harmful in high concentrations.

BIOLOGICAL HAZARDS

Question #3:
We're just serving food, what do we need to know about biology?

A. It's a new condiment.
   Hopefully not.

B. It's not located in the kitchen.
   Wrong.

C. Less than a bacteriologist and more than you might think!
   Move ahead.

Okay, maybe it's not necessary to know as much about biology as a bacteriologist or a physician, but it is important to know enough to keep yourself, the food you serve, and your customers safe. Knowing some background information about biological hazards will help put understanding behind the recommendations and regulations for food handling.

The organisms involved in foodborne illness have two different methods of causing problems: foodborne infection and foodborne intoxication.

Foodborne infection occurs when a person eats something with live germs that grow inside them. Heating foods to the correct temperature can kill these germs and make the food safe.

Foodborne intoxication occurs when a person eats something with bacteria-produced poisons (toxins) that won't be killed by heating. The agents causing these food infections and intoxications are bacteria, toxins, viruses, parasites, and fungi.

Bacteria

Question #4:
What goes from one to one million in seven short hours?

A. The number of things you have to do today.
   Seems like it.

B. Baby bunnies.
   Seems like it.

C. Reproduction-happy, illness-toting bacteria.
   Yep.

Bacteria are single-celled organisms that can cause foodborne illness in two ways: (1) They can infect foods themselves, by their presence in the food as they feed on it. (2) They can produce toxins, which make food hazardous, as they break down. Bacteria, under good conditions, can grow and divide quickly—each cell dividing into two approximately every 20 minutes. (See Fig. 1.1.)

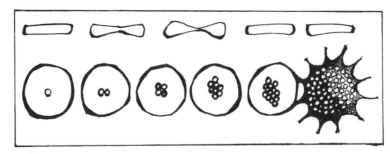

Fig. 1.1. Under the proper conditions, bacteria divide quickly, doubling every 20 minutes.

Good conditions for bacterial growth require

- Food — especially high-protein.
- Acidity — neutral to low acid.
- Temperatures — especially 40°–140°F. Ideal temperature is 90°–110°F, about body temperature.
- Time — more than four hours in the temperature range above.
- Oxygen.
- Moisture.

FAT TOM is an easy way to remember the conditions that can create food safety problems and need to be closely monitored.

When one or more of these six factors is present in a food product, creating the conditions for bacterial growth, that food product is a **potentially hazardous food.** (See Fig. 1.2.) Potentially hazardous foods therefore include meats; poultry; fish; soy-based foods; eggs; milk and milk products; cooked pasta, rice, potatoes, or beans; garlic-oil mixtures; raw fruits and vegetables; and raw seeds and sprouts. Some of these items surprise many people—it's not the mayonnaise (a higher-acid food) that is the problem on a buffet; rather, it is the moisture content and low acidity of the items that are put into the mayonnaise—potatoes, pasta, beans, etc. Some bacteria even produce spores that don't reproduce but can survive heating and cooling so that as conditions improve the spore's bacteria can become active again.

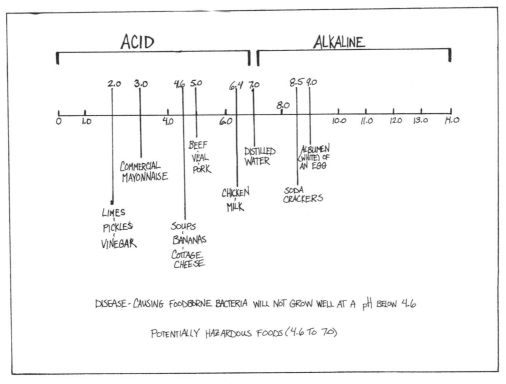

Fig. 1.2. Potentially hazardous foods (pH 4.6 to 7.0). Disease-causing bacteria will not grow well at a pH below 4.6.

Toxins

Toxins are substances that are produced by bacteria and are poisonous to other living tissue. Toxins and bacteria rarely cause any taste changes in food, so it may be almost impossible to tell if foods have been infected. Some toxins can come directly with the food supply. Some fish contain natural toxins; other fish, such as amber jacks and snapper, eat smaller fish infected with the natural toxin *ciguatoxin*. Tuna, bluefish, and mackerel can also produce toxins if held at an improper temperature. Toxins are not destroyed by cooking.

Viruses

Viruses are infectious agents, smaller than bacteria, that cannot reproduce on their own: they require a host cell. They do not reproduce in food, but they will withstand fluctuations in temperature. They appear in foods through poor food handling and poor hygiene techniques; this is the type of transmission that can be responsible for Hepatitis A infections.

Parasites

Parasites are organisms that live in or on another organism, usually causing the other organism harm. There are three types of parasites: protozoa, roundworms, and flatworms. Most commonly noted in food infections is the roundworm, *Trichinella spiralis,* found in pigs and wild game. Another roundworm is *Anisakis,* which is found in raw fish. These can be killed by proper cooking or freezing.

Fungi

Fungi are a group of single-celled organisms that are noted for their absence of chlorophyll. They include molds, mushrooms, and yeasts.

Molds become visible as they grow in number. They can cause food spoilage as well as produce toxins. Freezing prevents the growth of molds but does not kill organisms already present. Most foods with obvious signs of mold should be discarded. Exceptions include blue cheese, which has a natural mold running through it, and hard cheeses, which can have outside molds removed without any danger to the cheese underneath. Soft cheeses (cream cheese, cottage cheese, etc.), however, should be discarded if moldy.

Mushrooms are an edible fungus with the exception of poisonous varieties. The best protection against poisonous mushrooms is to buy them from a reputable supplier and wash thoroughly; **NEVER** incorporate handpicked mushrooms into quantity preparations.

Yeasts have many beneficial food applications. They can, however, spoil foods with a high sugar content, such as jelly or honey, by producing a bubbly alcohol smell. Foods with suspected yeast contamination should be thrown out.

STUDY QUESTIONS

1. Of the three hazards mentioned, which is the most harmful to people?

   A. Physical.
   B. Chemical.
   C. Biological.

2. Which of these would be a hazard in food?

   A. Bandage.
   B. Cherry pit.
   C. Fish bone.
   D. All of the above.

3. Which of these practices can help to reduce or minimize the growth of bacteria that cause foodborne infections?

   A. Allowing food to sit out at room temperature for the proper length of time.
   B. Heating foods quickly to the proper temperature.
   C. Leaving foods refrigerated at 50°F.

4. The best control measure for preventing bacterial growth is

   A. Controlling the length of time food is at 40°–140°F.
   B. Controlling the length of time canned food is stored on the shelf in the storeroom.
   C. Limiting the amount of food in the freezer.

EVALUATING YOUR FACILITY

1. What do the cooks at your facility do routinely to control physical hazards?

2. How could you improve your control of chemical hazards?

Chapter Two:
Foodborne Illnesses

LEARNING OBJECTIVES

After this chapter you should be able to

- List the major foodborne illnesses,
- Describe the causes of each foodborne illness, and
- Name the most important preventative measures.

The words "foodborne illness" can send shock waves through any facility, but especially those that have a large volume of customers that eat almost identically (schools, nursing facilities, congregate meal sites, etc.). Places with a fixed menu can infect a large number of people very quickly. Table 2.1 is designed to identify the major organisms that cause foodborne illness, detail the symptoms caused by each organism, and suggest how to prevent the occurrence of the associated foodborne illnesses.

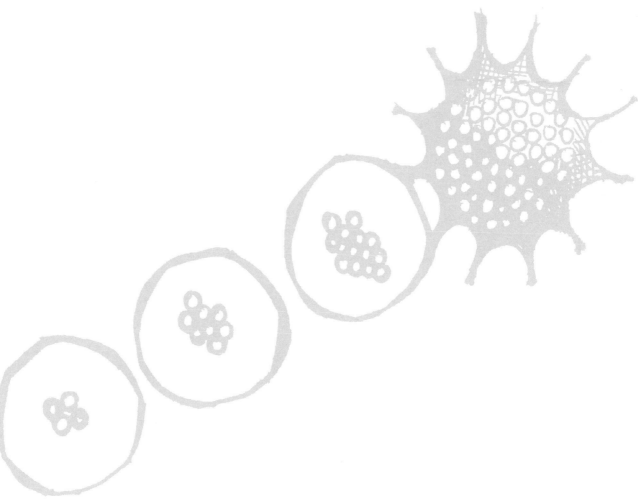

Table 2.1. Organisms and toxins that cause foodborne illness, the symptoms they cause, and how to prevent illness

ORGANISM, TOXIN, OR DISEASE	SYMPTOMS	TIME FRAME	CAUSES	TREATMENT	PREVENTION
			BACTERIA		
Salmonella	Fever, nausea, vomiting, diarrhea, cramps, headache	12–36 hours LASTS 4–7 days	Poultry, raw red meat, shellfish, eggs, dairy products, high-protein foods	2–4 million cases/year in the US Recover w/o treatment	Chill foods quickly Use pasteurized milk and egg products Avoid raw/cooked cross-contamination Sanitize equipment properly
E. coli O157:H7	Severe diarrhea, cramps, dehydration, nausea, malaise	12–24 hours LASTS 5–10 days	Unpasteurized milk, raw/rare ground beef, contaminated water—in foreign countries	Antidiarrheal medication Serious cases can require dialysis and blood transfusions	Caution when traveling Cook meat medium to well done (160°F or above) Drink municipal or bottled water Drink pasteurized milk
Vibrio vulnificus	Sudden chills, fever, nausea, vomiting, blood poisoning, and possibly death (in persons with weak immune systems) Septicemia 50% of the time, gastroenteritis, wound infection	Within 16 hours	Clams, oysters, crab—most common when served raw		If there is any underlying disease or illness DO NOT eat raw seafood

ORGANISM, TOXIN, OR DISEASE	SYMPTOMS	TIME FRAME	CAUSES	TREATMENT	PREVENTION
			BACTERIA		
Staphylococcus aureus	Severe vomiting, diarrhea, cramps, prostration	2–4 hours LASTS 2–3 days	Caused by enterotoxins. Meat products, egg products, pasta, sauces, potatoes, cream fillings, dairy products (all moist) Usually contaminated after cooking—poor hygiene techniques	Recover w/o treatment	Keep hot food hot and cold food cold Wash hands
Campylobacter	Fever, headache, muscle pain, diarrhea, stomach pain, nausea, fatigue Complications can include meningitis, urinary tract infection	2–10 days	Raw milk, contaminated water, raw or undercooked meat or poultry		Destroyed by cooking and water treatment Avoid cross-contamination of cutting boards Wash hands Cook meats to 160°F
Listeria	Fever, fatigue, nausea, vomiting, diarrhea Complications can include meningitis, septicemia, pneumonia, endocarditis, or miscarriage Most susceptible are people over 60, newborns, and/or immune compromised people	Flu symptoms: 12 hours Complications: 1–6 weeks	Soft cheese, unpasteurized dairy products, undercooked poultry, deli food	Antibiotics	Very resistant Thorough cooking will destroy Wash raw fruits and vegetables Avoid cross-contamination

Table 2.1. (continued)

ORGANISM, TOXIN, OR DISEASE	SYMPTOMS	TIME FRAME	CAUSES	TREATMENT	PREVENTION
BACTERIA					
Typhoid (disease caused by bacteria)	Malaise, fever, headache, cough, loss of appetite, nausea, vomiting, constipation, slow pulse, enlarged spleen, rose spots on body	7–28 days / LASTS 1–8 weeks / Can reoccur	Feces and urine of infected persons / Most common in developing countries / High-protein foods, raw salads, milk, shellfish. Any foods that are handled w/o further cooking	Antibiotics	Immunization / Good hygiene practices / Cook foods thoroughly / When traveling use the "boil it, cook it, peel it, or forget it" rule
Shigella (known as "bacillary dysentery")	Cramps, fever, chills, diarrhea, urge to urinate, dehydration, fatigue, and (sometimes) blood in stool / Symptoms vary	7–48 hours / LASTS 5–6 days	Comes from intestinal tract of animals, polluted water / Transmitted by poor hygiene to moist, mixed foods, milk, beans, potatoes, tuna, shrimp, turkey, pasta salads, apple cider, poi, raw foods	Antibiotics	Good hygiene practices / Chill foods quickly / Cook thoroughly—sensitive to heat / Control flies

ORGANISM, TOXIN, OR DISEASE	SYMPTOMS	TIME FRAME	CAUSES	TREATMENT	PREVENTION
		SPORE-FORMING BACTERIA			
Bacillus cereus (2 types)	DIARRHEAL: diarrhea, cramps, nausea	6–15 hours LASTS 24 hours	Meats, milk, vegetables, fish	Runs its course	Heat destroys bacteria but will not kill the toxin
	EMETIC: nausea, vomiting	1/2–6 hours LASTS <24 hours	Rice, pasta, potatoes, sauces, soups, puddings		
Clostridium perfringens	Abdominal pain, cramps	8–22 hours LASTS 24 hours Necrotic enteritis often fatal but very rare	Temperature abuse of foods especially meats, meat products, gravies, institutional feedings with large quantities of food made up ahead Found in the intestine of humans and animals	Runs its course	Keep hot foods hot and cold foods cold Reheat leftovers to 165°F or more
Clostridium botulinum	Headache, vomiting, double vision, severe fatigue, breathing difficulties Can be fatal	12–36 hours	Improper canning of low-acid foods— sausage, meats, veggies, seafood	Antitoxin must be administered promptly Considered a foodborne outbreak with a single case	Destroyed by proper canning at 176°F for >10 minutes NO garlic in oil at room temperature Keep foods refrigerated

Table 2.1. (continued)

ORGANISM, TOXIN, OR DISEASE	SYMPTOMS	TIME FRAME	CAUSES	TREATMENT	PREVENTION
TOXINS					
Ciguatera	Weakness, nausea, vomiting, diarrhea, abnormal sensory phenomenon (hot feels cold and vice versa), numbness of mouth, sweats, dizziness, pain	2–5 hours LASTS 4–8 hours up to 1 week	Fish that have eaten toxic algae from the Pacific or Caribbean	Recover w/o treatment	NOT destroyed by cooking Avoid repeated eating Clean fish quickly Do not eat head or roe of reef fish Buy from a reputable supplier
Scombroid	Dizziness, headache, nausea, flushing, itching, palpitations, cramps, diarrhea	Minutes to 2 hours LASTS 8–12 hours	Spoiling fish, especially tuna, mahimahi, albacore, sardines, and anchovies	Antihistamines	Clean and cook fish thoroughly Purchase and use quickly

ORGANISM, TOXIN, OR DISEASE	SYMPTOMS	TIME FRAME	CAUSES	TREATMENT	PREVENTION
			ENTEROVIRUS		
Hepatitis A (disease caused by enterovirus)	Fever, malaise, nausea, loss of appetite, fatigue, abdominal discomfort, jaundice, bile in urine Severity increases with age	10–50 days (depending on amount consumed) LASTS weeks to months	Water and shellfish from polluted/infected water are the most common sources Cross-contamination due to poor hand washing Ready-to-eat foods—cold cuts, donuts, sandwiches, milk, iced drinks—are often involved due to employee handling		Cook foods thoroughly Use good hygiene practices—WASH hands

Table 2.1. (continued)

ORGANISM, TOXIN, OR DISEASE	SYMPTOMS	TIME FRAME	CAUSES	TREATMENT	PREVENTION
			PARASITES[a]		
Trichinosis (disease caused by a parasite)	Nausea, vomiting, diarrhea, abdominal pain, excessive sweating, thirst, chills, skin lesions, weakness, prostration, edema of eyes, fever, muscle pain, difficulty breathing, toxemia, diseased heart muscle	4–28 days	Undercooked pork, wild game	Prescription drugs	COOK meat thoroughly until pork is white inside—above 155°F AVOID cross-contamination by washing anything raw meat has contacted. Wash and sanitize grinders, utensils, cutting boards
Cryptosporidium	Diarrhea, nausea, cramps, fever	LASTS 7–14 days	Fecally contaminated water or food Fecally contaminated environmental surfaces	No treatment available	NEVER drink water from lakes, swimming pools, or other untreated areas

[a]Parasites are dependent on a living host, i.e., an animal.

The bottom line for preventing foodborne illness is that appropriate food temperatures and good personal hygiene cannot be overemphasized. These are the key aspects to serving safe food.

If, however, the question of foodborne illness should arrive in your facility, remain calm. Typically, state agencies will investigate any reported foodborne illnesses based on confirmation from a stool sample and information given to them by the sickened individuals. As inspectors arrive at your facility be as helpful as possible by providing the information they require. Frequently requested items include schedules, recipes, heating and cooling procedures, and samples of food products in question if they are still available. Be cooperative, but do not answer questions from the media until the investigation is complete.

STUDY QUESTIONS

1. In order for a foodborne illness to be confirmed, it must
    A. Happen to lots of people.
    B. Occur only during the summer months of the year.
    C. Be confirmed through laboratory analysis.

2. *Salmonella* bacteria are transmitted through
    A. Infected pork.
    B. Infected beef.
    C. Infected poultry.

3. Trichinosis, which is found in pork, is which type of organism?
    A. Virus.
    B. Bacteria.
    C. Parasite.

4. *E. coli* bacteria are associated with what food and need to be cooked to what temperature to be killed?
    A. Ground beef, 155°F.
    B. Chicken, 165°F.
    C. Egg, 145°F.

5. Staph bacteria are transmitted through humans. What is the best control measure?
    A. Keep foods refrigerated.
    B. Proper and frequent hand-washing by food handlers.
    C. Proper and frequent hand-washing by customers.

6. Hepatitis is a disease caused by a virus. It is transmitted through

   A. Infected water.
   B. Dirty pans and utensils.
   C. Undercooked pork.

EVALUATING YOUR FACILITY

1. To what temperature do you routinely cook ground beef?

2. What are the most common factors in foodborne illness?

Chapter Three:

Preparation and Service of Safe Food

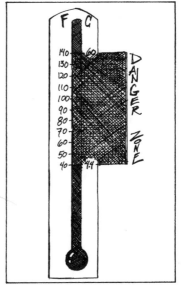

LEARNING OBJECTIVES

After reading this chapter you will be able to

- Identify the temperatures of the "danger zone,"
- Understand proper purchasing methods,
- Identify guidelines for refusing specific food items,
- Discuss proper storage of all food and non-food items,
- Name the most important aspect of personal hygiene,
- Explain cross-contamination,
- Identify acceptable thawing techniques,
- Name the "cook to" temperatures of potentially hazardous foods,
- Identify proper service methods, and
- Identify critical control points in a foodservice operation.

Question #5:
What is the single most important aspect of food safety?

A. Looking both ways before crossing the kitchen.
   A good idea but wrong.

B. Locking the lox.
   Wrong and a bad pun.

C. Temperatures.
   Yes. Put the safety ribbon here.

Throughout the food production chain (menu planning → purchasing → receiving → storage → preparation → service and holding of food products), **temperature** is the one element that remains a critical factor all along the way. Time/temperature abuse is the number one reason for foodborne illness. The range of temperatures that is most hazardous is 40°–140°F. It is in this range that bacteria have the best opportunity to grow and reproduce. To reduce the likelihood of bacterial growth, it is important to get foods through the "**Danger Zone**" of 40°–140°F (see Fig. 3.1) as quickly as possible by rapid chilling or rapid heating. Let us examine proper procedures for preventing foodborne illness at each point in the food production chain.

Fig. 3.1. Temperature danger zone where bacteria grow fastest is 40°–140°F.

keep hot food hot, keep cold food cold

MENU PLANNING

It's 6 p.m. and you open the refrigerator for dinner; you find ketchup, dill pickles, and some funny-smelling ground beef. So much for delicious. By planning ahead we are able to serve our customers (and ourselves) the best meals possible. Menu planning not only allows us to offer a variety of foods but also lets us use our refrigeration and cooking equipment appropriately. Planning ahead lets us purchase the right amount of each ingredient and allows us adequate storage space when it arrives. Menu planning makes it possible to look at preparation methods and equipment usage to produce high-quality foods maintained at the appropriate temperatures. This preplanning also gives us time to think about holding methods and potential plans for leftovers.

PURCHASING

Purchasing food for a facility is an important first step in the food-safety process. Foods must be purchased from reliable foodservice vendors. It is also important to have a written menu from which to make purchasing decisions. Items should be purchased in quantities and should be of a quality to match menu needs as well as storage capabilities. Order in quantities that allow for adequate airflow—especially through refrigerated and frozen storage.

It is a good idea over the course of business to tour supplier facilities to see their practices firsthand. This not only lets us appreciate their systems and difficulties but also allows us to look at their sanitation and food-handling practices. It is also a good idea to spell out your requirements in writing with regard to as many products as possible. This will lower the chance of refusals at delivery time for improper quality.

RECEIVING

The delivery man is here...there is something in the oven...quick, sign the papers...we'll get to it later. Unfortunately, scenes like this happen all the time. But receiving food products should be taken much more seriously. Specific times should be set up with vendors for product delivery. Time must be set aside in someone's schedule to check items in. This person must also be given the knowledge and authorization to decide whether or not a product must be refused. Provided in the following sections are guidelines for checking various classes of food products when they are received.

Frozen Foods Guidelines

All frozen foods need to be checked for temperature. Signs of thawing (wet, dripping packaging) or thawing and refreezing (frost, large ice crystals) are reasons to refuse delivery for both food-safety and food-quality reasons. These foods may be or may have been in the temperature danger zone for an extended period, allowing the growth of bacteria. The temperature of frozen products should be 0°F or below; test this by opening a case and inserting a thermometer between packages.

Shelf Life

Although shelf life varies with the product, a good rule of thumb is to keep things no longer than six months to prevent quality deterioration. Do not thaw and refreeze items: safety and quality become too questionable.

Dairy Products Guidelines

Buy only pasteurized milk or products made from pasteurized milk. Randomly check the temperature of different products as they arrive. Refuse products that are too warm (above 40°F). Check expiration dates on products, and refuse any that are outdated.

Shelf Life

Depending on the size of the facility and how often deliveries occur, maintain no more than a seven-day supply. Make sure dates on products will clear the time frame of the next delivery.

Meat and Poultry Guidelines

Buy items in the amounts needed as close to preparation time as possible; this practice reduces the need to rehandle or freeze extra portions. All meats and poultry products must be USDA inspected or have the equivalent state inspection stamp (most state stamps are in the shape of the state) (see Fig. 3.2). Check the temperature of the products and refuse any that are too warm (above 40°F), slimy, gray in color, or have an off odor. Additionally, the grade is an indication of the quality and palatability of the meat. Suppliers must be able to supply written proof that the meat is government inspected. Check pork at a point where the bone and flesh meet and smell for off odor. Fresh poultry should be packed on ice in cases that are self draining, so the poultry doesn't sit in its own bloody water.

 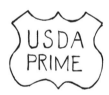 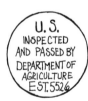

Fig. 3.2. USDA meat and poultry inspection labels.

Shelf Life

Poultry and ground or cut-up meats should be used in two days. Larger solid cuts of meat can last four to five days. **Modified atmosphere packaging (MAP)** is a technique that reduces the amount of oxygen in the package; this oxygen reduction will extend the shelf life of a product. Care should always be taken not to cut or tear the packaging of these products.

Fish and Seafood Guidelines

Fish and seafood must come from suppliers approved by the Interstate Certified Shellfish Shipper's List; this is to ensure that the supply is from unpolluted waters. This information can be on the box or a tag. Always check the temperature of fresh fish, refusing any fish that is too warm or slimy, has gills sticking close to the body, sunken eyes, or lack of springiness to the flesh (a push of a finger leaves an imprint), or has a strong fish odor. A 90-day file of shellfish identification tags must be kept after clams, mussels, and oysters have been received.

Shelf Life
Fish and seafood should be used in one to two days.

Egg Guidelines

Buy only government-inspected grade AA or A eggs. The FDA shield should appear on the carton of whole eggs. All pasteurized egg products should have a USDA inspection stamp (see Fig. 3.3). The proper temperature is 40°F or less. Check frozen egg products for signs of thawing, and refuse they if they are not frozen solid. Use pasteurized egg products for any item that does not get heated above 140°F.

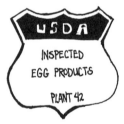 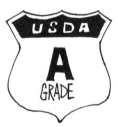

Fig. 3.3. USDA egg inspection labels.

Shelf Life
Use-by dates must be on the outside of each carton (no more than 30 days from the packing date). Use thawed egg products in three days. Store all eggs away from foods with strong odors such as fish, cabbage, and onions.

Produce Guidelines

Buy produce in quantities that will be used before items have a chance to spoil. Always check produce carefully for bruising or spoilage and refuse produce with any signs of decay. Buy from a reputable source.

Prepared Foods Guidelines

Premade salads, soups, sauces, entrees, etc. must be checked for maintenance of appropriate temperature (40°F or below). Check for any signs of damage to the containers (such as cracked lids, broken seals, and bulges or slits in the packaging) and refuse products as necessary. Check each product for use-by dates and refuse anything that expires within three days.

Dry Goods Guidelines

Check for and refuse any dented, leaking, or bulging cans. Refuse any product that does not have a label or whose edges appear to be rusted. NEVER use anything that has been home canned. Ultrapasteurized foods that are aseptically packaged can be maintained in a dry storage area until opened and then must be held appropriately under refrigeration.

STORAGE

Once the receipt of foods is complete, foods should NOT be allowed to sit on the dock or receiving area for half the day. Put food supplies away immediately—frozen and refrigerated products first. Do not overpack a refrigerator or freezer. If refrigeration is a problem (and who ever really has enough?), consider dividing deliveries into more days.

When storing items, allow for airflow around the product. Do not use trays or paper on shelves, since they block the airflow. Storage areas must be kept clean so that no off odors are picked up by the food. Do not use storage freezers to cool hot foods; this warms up the frozen products, causing thaw/refreeze damage. Wrap all foods in moisture-proof materials. Label and date anything that has been remove from its original container Remove staples, strapping, or other fasteners from boxes.

DO NOT STORE RAW PRODUCTS OVER COOKED OR READY-TO-EAT ITEMS. This is an easy way to avoid one product contaminating another (**cross-contamination**). Keep raw meats on the bottom shelves in pans to catch any blood or juices. In storage areas, keep food products separated from potentially hazardous items (pesticides, soaps, etc.). Store all foods at least six inches off the floor for good air circulation and reduced contact with moisture. Maintain a cool, low-humidity room (70°F with 50 percent humidity) for maximum storage life. See Figure 3.4.

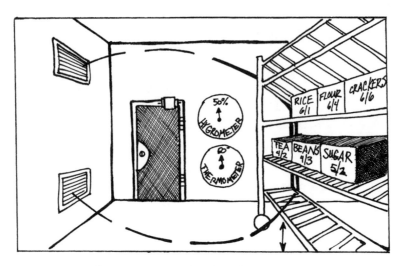

Fig. 3.4. Leave adequate space around products for good ventilation. Keep all products at least six inches off the floor.

Finally, rotate stock. These two very simple words, although important, are often hard to put into practice. The laws of human nature say to follow the path of least resistance; this means using what just came in. But the laws of safe food handling suggest something else: **First In, First Out** (better known as FIFO). Use up what is already in the refrigerator, freezer, or on the shelf before using new items. This will ensure that the products are used up quickly and nothing sits around waiting for bacteria to grow. Any product that comes in damaged or dented must be placed in a separate, designated area for return and/or credit.

PREPARATION

Now we're cookin'! The preparation phase of food production is the major source of foodborne errors. This is the place foods spend the most time and are exposed to the most hazards. This is a critical safety phase. Personal hygiene, culinary techniques, and cooking methods are all factors that will affect the final product safety outcome.

Personal Hygiene

Question #6, part a:
What are the three most important things to remember when buying a house?

A. Location, location, location.

Question #6, part b:
What are the three most important things to remember about personal hygiene and foodservice?

A. Wash your hands, wash your hands, wash your hands.

Hand-washing cannot be overemphasized. The next thought after "Wash your hands" might be, "Wear Gloves, wear gloves, wear gloves." However, although gloves are a great asset to food service, especially when handling foods that will remain raw (such as salads, fruits, deli meats, or desserts) or as protection over a bandage, they should never be mistaken for the answer to sanitation. Gloves are only as clean as what they touch. So if a person wearing gloves rubs his nose and then resumes working, the food is just as susceptible to new bacteria as if he had done the same thing with an ungloved hand.

Good hygiene practices must remain in place regardless of the use of disposable gloves. Every time a staff member leaves the kitchen, uses the restroom, works with raw product, takes a break, or touches something dirty, a thorough hand-washing must be completed. A thorough hand-washing requires the application of an antibacterial soap and a minimum 20-second rubbing of the hands together, working between the fingers and up over the wrists, followed by thorough rinsing and drying with a disposable towel or forced air. (A 20-second wash is approximately equivalent to singing one chorus of "Happy Birthday to You" at normal speed.) Then shut the water off with a paper towel. Still using the paper towel or a foot pedal, open the garbage and discard the towel (see Fig. 3.5).

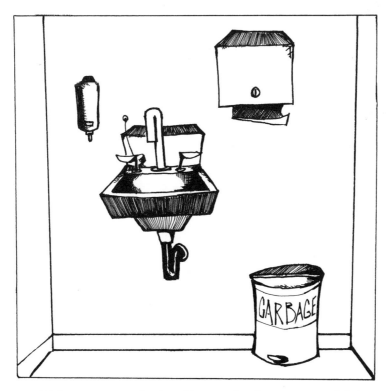

Fig. 3.5. Step up to proper hand-washing: a squirt of soap, water, work lather between fingers, over palms, and up wrists (humming "Happy Birthday"!), rinse, dry hands, turn off water with towel, step on garbage pedal, toss towel.

Other aspects of personal hygiene that are important to a foodservice operation include good grooming; a daily shower/bath, deodorant, and clean clothes are a must. Hair should be clean and restrained (by a hairnet, cap, etc.) to meet local inspection codes. Fingernails should be short, unpolished, and clean. No artificial fingernails should be worn in the foodservice environment. Again, jewelry should be kept to a minimum so it won't get caught in machinery or fall into a food product.

Staff should not eat while on duty: food and drinks can be too easily spilled into another food product. Product sampling, however, must be done as part of production process, either with disposable utensils or with enough silverware to allow for single-bite samplings. To taste, put a small bite on a dish, step away from the product (so nothing drips back into the main product), and use a utensil to sample the product. Discard disposable utensils; send others to the dishmachine. Use a new utensil for each tasting.

There should be no coughing or sneezing over or near food products. Staff needs to be encouraged to report any illnesses to a supervisor.

Culinary Techniques

As food is prepared, several items come into play that have the potential to interfere with the safety of our foods. Common to many of these items is the possibility of **cross-contamination**, which is the transfer of harmful microorganisms from infected items (hands, other contaminated foods, food contact surfaces, utensils, cleaning items, etc.) to a food product. Precautions for avoiding cross-contamination and growth of contaminating organisms are presented below.

COUNTERTOPS

Before any preparations can begin, the work surface must be sanitized. Wipe the area down with a santizing solution. Do not put food storage boxes or crates on the counter; if this is unavoidable, resanitize the area to avoid cross-contamination.

CUTTING BOARDS

Avoid the use of wood cutting boards in a facility. Wood acts as a host for many bacteria and odors. If wood is used in a bakery area, select a nontoxic hardwood such as maple. Thick plastic cutting boards are the preferred option.

Technique: Never use a cutting board for more than one item without washing and sanitizing. Never place a cooked item on a cutting board with raw product.

Safety Precaution: Place a piece of plastic washable matting between the table and cutting board to prevent the board from sliding. Replace cutting boards that are severely scratched to prevent any potential contamination.

KNIVES

Always use a knife for a single purpose. A knife must then be washed and sanitized before reuse.

Technique: Never slice through anything dirty that will be exposed to the item (for example, never cut through a dirty melon—the melon must be cleaned first so that none of the outside dirt is dragged through to the interior flesh).

Safety Precaution: NEVER drop a dirty knife into a dish sink or other water basin for someone else to clean. Always keep knives in plain sight of other staff.

SCOOPS/LADLES/TONGS

Technique: Use a scoop on one single product. Scoops must then be cleaned and sanitized. After cleaning scoops, a check should always be made for any stray particles by moving the sliding curve of a scoop back and forth. Do not allow the handles of any utensil to come into direct food contact. Keep the serving end in the product when not in use.

THAWING

Technique: The best way to thaw things is overnight in a refrigerator. When that amount of time is not available, items must be thawed under cool running water (below 70°F). Products can also be thawed as part of the natural cooking process, if appropriate to the recipe. Microwave ovens can also be used safely when the product is going to be immediately cooked further. Follow manufacturer guidelines for thawing. These methods will help to maintain the product temperature outside the temperature danger zone. NEVER thaw anything on a countertop or under hot water.

MIXING

Technique: To properly mix products, have items chilled or heated as appropriate to keep out of the temperature danger zone (for example, for chicken salad, have the chicken and the salad dressing well chilled prior to mixing). Do not let potentially dangerous foods come to room temperature.

TIMING

Timing is everything, especially for food, and should be limited to two hours of preparation time without being heated or chilled. If you are called away from a product, the item should be wrapped and refrigerated until preparation can begin again.

Cooking Methods

So now all these dishes are prepared and it is time to cook or chill the product. Here's how to do it.

HEATING

Whatever heating method is chosen (baking, grilling, sautéing, etc.), it needs to be done quickly enough to minimize the amount of time a product stays in the temperature danger zone (40°–140°F). Safe internal temperatures for selected cooked products are shown in Table 3.1.

Table 3.1. Safe internal temperatures of selected cooked products

PRODUCT	INTERNAL TEMPERATURE (°F)
Eggs	145
Beef roasts	145
Fish	145
Pork, ham, sausage	155
Ground meats	155
Poultry	165
Game meats	165
Stuffings for meats, fish or pasta	165

THERMOMETERS

A word or two about thermometers is in order here. NEVER use glass thermometers; it is too easy for them to break, releasing potentially hazardous mercury. Select thermometers that have a short response time and are accurate within 2°F. Appropriate choices include bimetallic, digital, and thermocouple thermometers.

Bimetallic thermometers, with easy-to-read numbering, have a sensor tip for reading temperatures located on the first inch of the stem. The most accurate reading comes 15 seconds after the sensor stops moving. These stem thermometers (see Fig. 3.6) are the most common. Calibrate thermometers frequently to prevent inaccuracies. To calibrate a stem thermometer, insert it into an ice bath, wait for the needle to stop, then use a small wrench to adjust the temperature to 32°F (0°C).

Digital thermometers measure temperatures either through a sensing tip or a pad, then provide a digital readout. A thermocouple uses a sensor tip as well and provides a digital readout at the press of a button. These thermometers (see Fig. 3.6) are accurate for a wide range of temperatures and need less calibration than stem thermometers but are much more expensive. If the temperature is inaccurate on a digital or thermocouple thermometer, change the battery and retest.

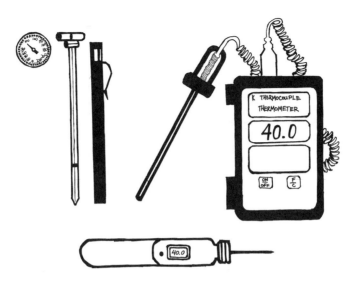

Fig. 3.6. Bimetallic (left), digital (bottom), and thermocouple thermometers (right).

MICROWAVING

This method of heating can be used, but add 25°F to the internal temperatures listed above. Stir or rotate the product during the microwaving process and allow the products to stand two minutes after cooking is complete to distribute heat throughout.

CHILLING

Once a product has been made and/or served it needs to pass back through the temperature danger zone quickly. The product should be cooled to 71°F within two hours and to 40°F within the four hours after that. So within six hours the hot product should have passed completely through the temperature danger zone. But the faster a product is cooled the better. This can be done by placing items in an ice bath; transferring foods into shallow pans no deeper than two to three inches (studies have shown that the temperature in a deep stock pot can still be at 120°F after six hours in a refrigerator); and/or using temperature reduction devices (i.e., ice-filled plastic tubes used to reduce the internal temperature of products). All refrigerator shelving should be slotted so that cool air can circulate quickly around the product: do not line shelves with pans or foil. NEVER let products cool on a counter.

For most facilities two final words of advice may be easier said than done: DON'T OVERCROWD.

HOLDING

Keeping hot food hot and cold food cold is a tricky foodservice task. To minimize holding times (which typically increases quality), as often as possible make food in small batches and serve immediately. For those products where small batches aren't possible, frequently stir or baste to keep temperature well distributed. NEVER use holding equipment (steam tables, crock pots, heated transportation carts) to cook a product. Items that are to be held cold should be refrigerated or packed in ice. Check temperatures frequently on product chilling or reheating to maintain appropriate temperatures—below 40°F or above 140°F.

SERVICE

Whether it is white glove, five-star service; a cafeteria tray line; or pass-the-plate home-style service, some basic rules apply. First and foremost is good personal hygiene. Hand-washing and good grooming are a must. Use clean and sanitized service pieces when providing the customer with any food item. Never touch food contact portions of dishes, glassware, or flatware (the rim of a cup, the center of a plate, the tines of a fork, the inside of a soup bowl, etc.). Fingers should only touch the base of a glass or mug (see Fig. 3.7), the saucer or handle of a cup, the rim of a plate, or the handles of flatware.

For self-service areas (such as salad bars), provide adequate plates to allow customers to take a new plate on a return trip; prohibit the reuse of used dishes.

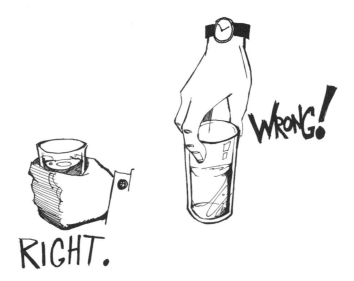

Fig. 3.7. Right and wrong ways to hold a glass or mug when serving.

REHEATING

Question #7:
What is the best advice to give when a busload of high school students never shows up—leaving you with 2000 pounds of leftover food?

A. "Throw it out, who really cares about food costs"?
    Not if you want a job tomorrow.

B. "Mix it all together, top with cheese, and use it as tomorrow's Chef's Surprise"?
    Creative but wrong.

C. "Chill it quickly in shallow pans and then reheat to a temperature above 165°F"?
    Smart.

Reheat products thoroughly to above 165°F. Do not mix reheated products with fresh. Discard any unused portion after it has been reheated once. NEVER use holding equipment to reheat foods.

HACCP

CDC, FDA, USDA, W, X, Y, and Z...the government makes great use of letters! HACCP (HaSip, as it is phonetically pronounced) is an acronym for Hazard Analysis Critical Control Points. This program, which was first developed by Pillsbury Company for NASA, is a scientific system designed to prevent food-safety hazards. This is done with appropriate controls during each stage of the food handling and production flow. Through **task analysis**, the system identifies specific points (**critical control points** or CCPs) at each stage where safeguards can be used to prevent contamination. See Table 3.2 for control points and safeguard suggestions.

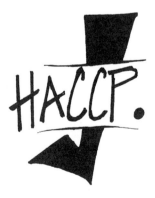

Fig. 3.8. HACCP logo.

Table 3.2. HACCP critical control points (CCPs) and suggested safeguards at each CCP

Source
Using a reputable supplier.
↓

Delivery
Refusing unacceptable products.
Checking all deliveries.
↓

Storage
Storing perishable foods properly.
First in, first out.
↓

Cooking
Thawing foods properly.
Cleaning and sanitizing of work areas, equipment, and serviceware.
Avoiding cross-contamination.
Cooking potentially hazardous foods to the appropriate temperature to destroy bacteria.
Using good personal hygiene.
↓

Holding
Holding hot food above 140°F.
Holding cold food below 40°F.
↓

Serving
Using clean disposable gloves to handle ready-to-eat items.
Avoiding cross-contamination.
Using good personal hygiene.
↓

Chilling
Chilling foods to 71°F in two hours and to 40°F in four more hours.
Avoiding cross-contamination.
Using good personal hygiene.
↓

Reheating
Reheating foods to at least 165°F.
No mixing of old and new food products.

These safeguards are great checkpoints, and in some informal way we are probably doing all or some of these items. A HACCP program pulls all these things together to more formally look at our procedures and operations. From this information, monitoring and corrective action plans are established, making solutions and responsibilities much more clear. The monitoring systems include time and temperature logs, visual observations of food inspection and preparation, sensory evaluations, and chemical tests to measure pH or viscosity.

Much of this information can be easily included in recipes, cleaning procedures, and sanitation checklists. For example, in a recipe that calls for cut-up raw chicken and chopped vegetables the HACCP checkpoints would include

- Cut chicken and vegetables on separate, clean cutting boards;
- Cook to an internal temperature of 165°F or more;
- Check holding temperature and reheat if it drops to 140°F or below;
- Cool leftovers quickly in a two-inch shallow pan; and
- Reheat leftovers to at least 165°F and do not reuse more than once.

All these points can be easily added to the methods portion of a recipe to emphasize the importance of these hazards. At any of these checkpoints, if the product does not meet the standard (for example, the holding temperature falls below 140°F), then corrective action needs to take place immediately (such as reheating the product to 165°F). A HACCP worksheet with corrective action guidelines to follow can be a great safety net when working with potentially hazardous foods. A worksheet is included as Appendix 1.

Information about food safety has been recently condensed for public use. The campaign—Fight BAC!—consists of public service announcements on safe food preparation. The four key messages are

1. Wash hands and surfaces often.
2. Prevent cross-contamination.
3. Cook foods to proper temperatures.
4. Refrigerate foods promptly.

These four points are key factors in food preparation and prevention of foodborne illness at work and at home.

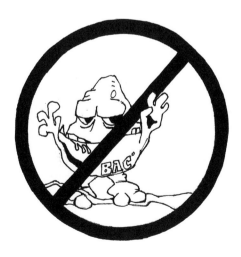

Fig. 3.9. Fight BAC logo.

STUDY QUESTIONS

1. What is the temperature danger zone?

    A. The temperature at which bacteria grow most rapidly.
    B. The temperature at which food is the safest.
    C. The best temperature for storing foods.

2. What is the range of the temperature danger zone?

    A. 41°–150°F.
    B. 45°–120°F.
    C. 40°–140°F.

3. At which stage do you have the most control of the temperature danger zone?

    A. Menu planning.
    B. Receiving.
    C. Preparation and holding.

4. When receiving fresh poultry, what is the proper temperature?

    A. 40°F or above.
    B. 45°F or below.
    C. 40°F or below.

5. Always buy your poultry and dairy products from?

    A. The farmer down the road.
    B. A reputable supplier.
    C. The black market.

6. Use a pasteurized egg product in which recipe?

    A. Banana cream pie.
    B. Ham and cheese omelet.
    C. Hard fried eggs.

7. Which of these items are potentially hazardous?

    A. Eggs, beans, custard pie, turkey.
    B. Flour, dry beans, unopened canned gravy.
    C. Dry noodles, powdered eggs, powdered milk.

8. Which of these canned goods may be used?

   A. A can with no label.
   B. A can with a sharp dent in the side.
   C. A can with only one end bulging.

9. To ensure FIFO is working, label and date all products, then

   A. Use most current dated products first.
   B. Use everything before you have to date it.
   C. Use oldest dated products first.

10. What is the only substitution for good hand-washing?

    A. A glove.
    B. A sanitizing gel.
    C. There is no substitution for good hand-washing.

11. Which of these tasks are examples of cross-contamination?

    #1: Cutting up raw chicken on a cutting board followed by cutting up lettuce on the same cutting board.

    #2: Stirring raw ground beef with a spoon and then using the same spoon to clean seeds from a cantaloupe.

    #3: First dicing an onion for soup, then using the same knife and cutting board to dice up raw turkey for the same soup.

    A. 1, 2, and 3 are all cross-contamination.
    B. 1 and 2.
    C. 2 and 3.

12. What is a proper way to thaw foods?

    A. Under cool running water.
    B. In a microwave oven as long as the item is completely cooked in an approved method after being thawed.
    C. Under refrigeration for 24–48 hours.
    D. All of the above.

13. What is the safest, most accurate thermometer to measure cold food temperatures?

   A. A candy thermometer.
   B. A glass-stemmed thermometer.
   C. A bimetallic-stemmed thermometer.

14. Which methods are approved for chilling?

   #1: Reducing the mass to cool under refrigeration.

   #2: An ice bath.

   #3: Counter-top cooling method.

   A. 1, 2, and 3.
   B. 1 and 2.
   C. 2 and 3.

15. The correct reheat temperature is?

   A. 155°F.
   B. 160°F.
   C. 165°F.

16. HACCP (Hazard Analysis Critical Control Point) is?

   A. More letters to remember.
   B. Controls to make a point of analyzing.
   C. A system that identifies critical control points where safeguards can be used to prevent contamination.

EVALUATING YOUR FACILITY

1. Follow the production of a potentially hazardous food through your kitchen—how long was the product held in the temperature danger zone? What could be done to shorten that time?

2. What HACCP-type steps do you already use routinely to ensure your food is safe?

3. What is your hand-washing policy? Is it posted anywhere in the facility? Are new employees trained in proper hand-washing?

Chapter Four:
Cleaning and Sanitation

LEARNING OBJECTIVES

After this chapter you should be able to

- State the differences between "clean" and "sanitize,"
- List the factors affecting cleaning,
- Identify the types of cleaning chemicals,
- List the methods of sanitizing,
- Understand the chemical sanitizing options,
- Identify appropriate wash, rinse, and sanitize temperatures for different equipment, and
- List the steps in cleaning dishes and pots and pans.

Question #8:
What is the most fun a person can have in a day?

A. Being with people who adore you.
   Great choice if you can find them.

B. Winning the lottery (tax free).
   Another good answer, let's shop!

C. Washing and sanitizing work surfaces.
   Four words: you need better hobbies!

Maybe cleaning and sanitizing don't top the list of great things to do for fun. They do, however, top the list of great things to do for safe food. And since these two words are often used together, let's define them. **Cleaning** is the physical removal of dirt, trash, tarnish, stain, or other materials creating mess, clutter, or filth. It includes washing. **Sanitizing** is the process that reduces or eliminates bacteria and other microorganisms to levels that will not cause food spoilage. The sanitizing process use either high temperatures or chemical agents to kill the bacteria.

All food contact surfaces must be cleaned, rinsed, and sanitized prior to use.

CLEANING

Remove the dirt. This seems simple. There are, however, many factors that can affect or interfere with this simple cleaning process.

Physical Conditions

Whether the dirt is fresh, dried on, baked on, or soaked in will determine the specific cleaner, method, and time to be used.

Time

The longer a cleaner or scrubbing action is used on a surface, the better the cleaning will be.

Water

Water must be from a safe source and of the proper temperature. The higher the temperature, the quicker things dissolve, making cleaning easier and more thorough. Water pressure is also a factor—the more force or agitation used in the cleaning process the more likely dirt is to be removed.

Chemicals

All cleaners are chemical compounds designed to remove a particular dirt or mineral. Solubility (the ability to dissolve in another substance, such as water) is a factor in the choice of chemicals. Some dirt is water soluble (flour, starch, sugar), while other dirts are insoluble in water (margarine, animal fat, oils), and they require different conditions for removal. The pH of the dirt (very acidic to alkaline) will also influence the cleaning method used; acidic cleaners, for example, are used when aklaline cleaners don't work (on rust, tarnish, or lime deposits, for example). The best cleaners are stable, noncorrosive agents that are safe for the user and the surface. Common cleaning agents may include any of the following types:

DETERGENTS

Contain surfactant substances that alter surface tension, which allows the detergent to remove the soil. Detergents are easily rinsed. Concentrations, however, should ALWAYS be prepared according to the manufacturer's directions. Detergents work most efficiently at higher temperatures because as the water temperature goes up the water molecules are moving faster so the detergent is moving faster—and cleaning more efficiently. As the water temperature cools the detergent moves more slowly, so more is needed. Therefore, a continuous check on wash-water temperature is beneficial. Detergents are usually used to remove fresh dirt from surfaces; a stronger solution may be needed remove baked-on or greasy dirt or wax buildup from surfaces.

DEGREASERS

Degreasers are alkaline detergents that have an added grease-dissolving agent. These chemicals are used to clean grill and oven surfaces, oven racks, etc. These are very strong chemicals, and good safety precautions should be used. Adequate ventilation, eye protection, and gloves are a must when using these chemicals.

DE-LIMERS

De-limers are acidic cleaners to use where alkaline products aren't strong enough. These chemicals are used frequently to remove buildup from dishmachines. Safety precautions again must be followed.

ABRASIVES

Abrasives are cleaners that contain scouring agents to lift off heavy soils. These chemicals are used on floors and walls and on pans with baked/burnt-on dirt. Abrasives can scratch soft surfaces and are not recommended for Plexiglas, plastics, or stainless steel.

CHELATING AGENTS

Chelating agents are chemicals that help control mineral deposits by softening the water.

All chemicals MUST be stored away from food supplies and MUST have clearly readable labels. The kitchen is not a chemistry lab: NEVER mix chemicals together; they can become corrosive to equipment and/or emit toxic fumes harmful to people.

RINSING

Rinsing is a must on all food-contact surfaces to remove any cleaning solution residues. Warm water rinsing is most effective, but this temperature will vary depending on the equipment used. Rinsing must be thorough because detergent can raise the pH of sanitizing solutions and make them ineffective.

SANITIZING

Sanitizing a surface to make it food safe must be done prior to use, after each use, after interruption of service, and at regular intervals as appropriate. Sanitizing can be accomplished by one of two methods, heat or chemicals.

Heat

Temperatures above 165°F are needed to kill microorganisms. Water must be heated to and maintained at 180°F (or 170°F in some states) to be effective. This requires a booster heater or a heating element in the final rinse tank. Items must be immersed in the hot water for not less than 30 seconds. This method is effective for dishmachines. Heat sanitizing by immersion, however, is dangerous for pot and pan sinks due to skin contact with the hot water. It is also too difficult to maintain the high temperature for surface sanitizing.

Chemicals

Use of sanitizing chemicals, registered as pesticides by the FDA, is an effective sanitation method, but the chemicals MUST be used properly. If too little chemical is used it can be ineffective in killing microorganisms; if too much is used, the chemical can be considered harmful. Self-dispensing equipment that is routinely maintained is often the best method for using such chemicals. Chemicals are effective at much lower temperatures (75°–120°F) than those used for heat sanitizing, making things easier to handle. Immersion time is at least one minute in the three-compartment sink system. For the dishmachine, chemicals are introduced in the final rinse automatically and for the appropriate length of time. Table 4.1 shows various chemical sanitizing options and their benefits, drawbacks, and use requirements. As with any hazardous chemical, ALWAYS FOLLOW THE LABEL DIRECTIONS.

Table 4.1. Chemical sanitizing options

	CHLORINE	IODINE	QUATERNARY AMMONIUM
Benefits	Inexpensive	Nonirritating	Nonirritating
Drawbacks	Damages pewter, stainless steel, and silver plate Can leave an off odor	Noncorrosive	Noncorrosive
Concentration needs	50–100 ppm **MUST CHECK WITH A TEST STRIP**	12.5–25 ppm Water will be amber colored **MUST CHECK WITH A TEST STRIP**	200 ppm Hard water above 500 ppm can make quaternary ammonium less effective **MUST CHECK WITH A TEST STRIP**
Water pH	Must be below 8.0	Must be below 5.0	Works best at 7.0, but can work in both acidic and alkaine conditions
Water temperature	75°F	75°–120°F	75°F
Time needed to sanitize	At least 1 minute	At least 1 minute	At least 1 minute

Table 4.2 shows the minimum water temperatures needed to meet federal and state requirements throughout the wash, rinse, and sanitizing process.

Table 4.2. Minimum water temperature for dishmachine and pot and pan sinks

CYCLE	LOW-TEMPERATURE DISHMACHINE	HIGH-TEMPERATURE DISHMACHINE	THREE-COMPARTMENT SINK, MANUAL POTS AND PANS
Prewash	80°–110° F	80°–110° F	75°–120°F
Wash	120°F	150°F one tank, stationary 150°F multi-tank conveyor 160°F single-tank conveyor 120°F	
Rinse	75°–120°F	180°–195°F	75°–120°F
Sanitize	75°–120°F, chemical	180°F	75° 120°F, chemical 170°–180°F, heat

METHODS

Every facility needs to have cleaning schedules and systems in place to ensure that cleaning is done routinely and correctly. Products will vary, but the methods should remain the same.

Equipment, Utensil Storage, and Food Contact Surfaces

Step 1. Warm detergent water, a clean towel, rinse water, and a spray bottle of sanitizer should be gathered.

Step 2. At the beginning of each shift, counters and other food contact surfaces should be washed free of dirt. After each use, each piece of equipment should be TURNED OFF and washed free of noticeable dirt and spots. Abrasives and scrub pads should be used only on hard surfaces where scratching won't occur.

Step 3. The surface should be rinsed to remove any detergent residue.

Step 4. Surfaces should be sprayed or wiped with a sanitizing solution and allowed time to air dry.

Stationary Equipment

Permanent, nonrolling equipment needs to be at least six inches off the floor (on legs, a sealed masonry base, or wall mounted). Permanent countertop equipment must have at least four-inch legs or be completely sealed to the counter. Spaces around each piece of equipment should follow manufacturer's guidelines and allow for adequate cleaning. The same wash, rinse, sanitizing, and air dry methods apply.

Manual Pot and Pan Washing

Step 1. Each compartment of the three-compartment sink (see Fig. 4.1) is filled with water at the appropriate temperature.

Step 2. The appropriate amount of soap (following label directions) is added to the first tank. The appropriate amount of sanitizer is added to the third sink (following label directions) and is confirmed by a test strip. Automatic soap and sanitizer dispensers work well for providing consistent amounts of product to each tank.

Step 3. Items to be cleaned are stacked near the soap tank end of the sink. Every item is scraped clean of debris using a scraper or a high pressure sprayer. Then the item is placed in the soap tank. Wash towels, scratchers (if appropriate), and scrubbers can be used to clean any remaining soil or buildup off the item. NEVER drop knives into the sink for someone else to wash. Either establish a location to place dirty knives or make each person responsible for washing their own knives. Do not submerge or soak wooden cutting boards; they need to be washed with a stiff brush, rinsed, and sanitized after each use.

Step 4. Once the items have been wiped clean in the soap water, they must be rinsed to allow for maximum sanitation. Move the item from the soap tank to the water tank for rinsing. Submerge completely.

Step 5. Once rinsed, the item is placed in the third sink for sanitizing. Items must remain submerged in the sanitizing solution for at least one minute or as long as required by manufacturer guidelines.

Step 6. Items are then removed from the sanitizer and laid out to air dry: NEVER hand dry items. Allow enough time and space for items to dry completely. Once dried, with no signs of residue, the items can be put away appropriately. Items on shelves should be stored upside down.

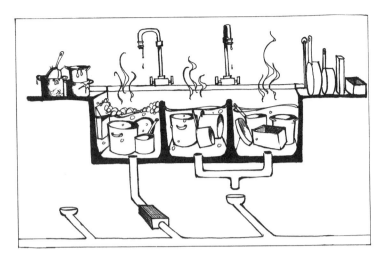

Fig. 4.1. Three-compartment sink work area for manual pot and pan washing. Note the air gap between the sinks and the drain.

Dishwashing by Machine

There are five elements that share equal responsibility for the overall effectiveness of a dish machine. These elements are time, water temperatures, chemicals, mechanical function, and operating procedures.

Step 1. Fill the water tanks of the machine. Turn on the tanks to allow them time to heat up. Check for adequate soap and sanitizer and refill as necessary.

Step 2. Presoak any dried-on foods, especially protein foods. Scrape excess food and paper products off dishes. Load appropriately into the dish-machine racks. DO NOT OVERLOAD the racks and do not surround smaller items by larger ones; both these procedures will make it very difficult for water to contact all the surfaces. Place the racks into a single unit machine or place on a conveyor type system and allow the cycle to run uninterrupted. Check the scrap baskets periodically and empty them as needed. Change the water every two hours.

Step 3. After the sanitizing portion of the cycle is completed, allow the dishes time to thoroughly air dry before putting them away. Always put away dishes with the rims of glasses turned down. Plates and dishes are also placed upside down on rubber-matted shelves or in a lowerator for later use.

Step 4. Spot-check the temperature of the booster heater (this applies to high-temperature machines) and run test strips through the machine to check for adequate sanitizing. Check for mineral deposits in the machine and use a de-limer as needed.

Table 4.3 provides a checklist of common dishmachine and pot and pan cleaning difficulties that can help target the source of a problem.

Table 4.3. Troubleshooting: possible causes of and solutions to dishmachine and pot and pan washing problems.

PROBLEM	POSSIBLE CAUSE	POSSIBLE SOLUTIONS
DISHMACHINE		
Coffee, tea stains	Wrong detergent	Use a detergent with chlorine in it.
Dirty dishes	Not enough detergent	Check soap dispensers.
	Not enough water	Check water levels, O-rings, spray-arm end caps.
	Wash temperature too low	Keep temperature close to 160°F.
	Inadequate wash and rinse time	Do not force dishes through a machine faster than the conveyor belt or automatic timer allows.
	Unclean equipment	Unclog spray nozzles to improve the spray pattern on the dishes. Check scrap baskets for debris.
	Too much water	Check the automatic fill— it may be stuck.
	Racking the dishes wrong	Do not overcrowd dishes. Keep all dishes going in the same direction. Do not "sandwich" small items between bigger items—water won't reach.
Film—white, cloudy film	Water hardness	Use water-softening agent. Check for water temperatures above the recommended ranges—water that is too hot can create a film.
	Final rinse	Check for water in the final rinse tank.
	Lime buildup in the machine	De-lime the machine to keep final rinse clear. Keep heating elements clean and free of buildup.

PROBLEM	POSSIBLE CAUSE	POSSIBLE SOLUTIONS
DISHMACHINE		
Foaming	Detergent	Change to a low-sudsing product.
	Food soil	Empty scrap baskets, prescrape all dishes.
Greasy film—lipstick, food grease	Low pH	Maintain adequate alkalinity to trap grease.
	Low water temperature	Check water temperature. High temperature is very important to break down fat.
	Dirty equipment	Check spray-arm nozzles. Change water in tanks.
Spotting	Rinse water hardness	Use a water softener.
	Rinse water temperature	Too high—dishes may be "flash" drying or too low— water may be drying on dishes instead of running off.
	Procedures	Check for a missing curtain before the final rinse tank. Allow time for dishes to dry completely before stacking.
Streaking	High pH	Use external treatment to reduce alkalinity. Check for a rinse additive to eliminate streaks.
	Dirty equipment	Check spray arms for adequate pressure. Check for adequate rinse water.
POTS AND PANS		
Dirty pots	Not enough detergent	Check dispenser or check the amount use manually with the number of gallons in the sink to see if it is appropriate.
Greasy film	Dirty water	Change water tanks: clean after they are drained and then refill.

From Table 4.3 it is clear that many dishmachine problems are the result of dirty equipment. Keeping the equipment clean will both increase the efficiency of the machine and its operators and maintain customer satisfaction.

Clean in Place

Clean-in-place equipment includes those items that are cleaned by running a cleaning agent through equipment (ice cream machines, self-cleaning ovens, and hood systems, for example). Manufacturer's directions for cleaning should be followed, and all food contact surfaces should be thoroughly cleaned.

Non—Food Contact Surfaces

This category includes such areas as floors, ceilings, and restrooms.

Step 1. Clear the area of any debris. Cover or remove any food products that might be in the way.

Step 2. Using a detergent, mop or wipe the area clean.

Step 3. Wring out mop or towel and rinse the cleaned area.

Step 4. For floor drains, wear rubber gloves. Remove the cover and clean out any trapped debris; replace the cover; then flush area with hot water followed by sanitizer.

Step 5. Replace any needed items (i.e., floor mats, toilet paper, hand towels, soap, etc.).

This step approach to cleaning and sanitizing—a sort of recovery program for cleanliness—is only as effective as its enforcement. Assignments need to be made to ensure that tasks are being completed on a routine basis. A daily sanitation walk-through by management staff is important for maintaining the cleanliness of the kitchen as well as for checking for potential food hazards and viewing food-handling techniques.

STUDY QUESTIONS

1. Which factors most positively affect the process of cleaning a pan?

   A. Light amount of pressure applied, cold water temperatures, plenty of de-limer.
   B. Good soaking time, contaminated water, twice the recommended amount of detergent.
   C. Proper solubility, adequate soak time, proper concentration of soap.

2. The proper cleaning cycle is

   A. Wash, rinse, towel dry.
   B. Rinse, wash, soak, dry on counter.
   C. Wash, rinse, sanitize, air dry.

3. To sanitize with HOT water in the final rinse tank, the water temperature needs to be

    A. 120°F for 10 minutes.
    B. 180°F for 30 seconds.
    C. 212°F for 10 seconds.

4. What is the proper temperature range for effective chemical sanitizing?

    A. 70°–125°F.
    B. 75°–120°F.
    C. 70°–120°F.

EVALUATING YOUR FACILITY

1. What are the problems you experience in your facility with clean dishes? What ways can these be troubleshot?

Chapter Five:
Safety

LEARNING OBJECTIVES

After this chapter you should be able to

- List the advantages of employee training,
- Identify items that should be in place for optimal safety conditions, and
- Understand Material Safety Data Sheets and their purpose.

Question #9:
What is the best way to address safety issues?

A. With a big stack of Incident Reports and a sharp pencil.
   Wrong.

B. Right after you hear your lead cook will be out for six weeks with a back injury and find out the costs of replacing him/her.
   So much for the labor budget.

C. Before there are problems.
   A safety pin for you.

Employee safety is a very important concern. Lost time due to work injury is harmful in several ways: the physical effects on the employee, the interruption of the work routine (i.e., job reassignments), increases in insurance costs, and so on. Therefore, it is most beneficial to address the needs of the staff early and provide the appropriate tools to do the work. This process includes providing

- A safety orientation for all new employees (no running, no dropping knives into dishwater, proper use of equipment, etc.).
- Inservice reminders.
- New-equipment training.
- Equipment in good working order (look for the Underwriters Laboratories, Inc., mark, shown in Fig. 5.1).
- Adequate carts in good repair for moving heavy items.
- Back braces for those employees who do heavy lifting.
- Nonskid floor matting in dishmachine and manual wash areas.
- Slicer guard(s) in working order and mesh gloves.
- Well-sharpened knives.
- An ample supply of pot holders (large ones intended for institutional use) and oven mitts.

■ Appropriate utensils for jobs (long-handled spatulas, step stools to reach high places, etc.).
■ Warning signs near hazardous equipment/conditions.
■ A well-stocked first aid kit.

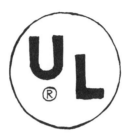

Fig. 5.1. The Underwriters Laboratories, Inc., seal on your equipment shows that the equipment has been tested for safety.

The Occupational Safety and Health Administration (OSHA) is the regulatory agency that monitors safety in the workplace. According to OSHA regulations every employee has the **right to know** what he/she is exposed to during the course of a work day. Therefore, all employees must be trained properly in using hazardous materials as well as be supplied with the appropriate materials for handling such items. The following should be available to every employee:

■ Clearly labeled products with directions for use.
■ A Material Safety Data Sheet (MSDS) for every hazardous compound used in the department. An MSDS contains the following information:

- The common and chemical names for the product
- Where the product is to be used
- How the product is to be used
- Hazards associated with use of the product (fire, poison, skin irritant, etc.)
- Protection required when using the product
- Emergency procedures for exposure to or spillage of the product
- How to properly store the product

■ Protective gloves, goggles, face masks, and aprons.
■ Spray hose.
■ Eye wash station.
■ Appropriate supplies—buckets, mops, brooms, dustpans, step stools to reach high places.
■ Training—NEVER let an employee use chemicals that are unfamiliar. Instruct employees on proper concentrations, appropriate uses, hazards, and the importance of never mixing chemicals together.

Every employee should know to report unsafe work practices to a supervisor. The supervisor then is responsible for taking corrective action to fix the unsafe condition—through employee education, changing procedures, and/or purchasing new equipment.

The bottom line about safety is, "Think of it first and then it won't be a problem."

STUDY QUESTIONS

1. To ensure safety in a kitchen, you should

   #1: Run instead of walk.

   #2: Use well-stacked milk crates to climb high.

   #3: Use a wet towel to lift a hot pan.

   A. 1, 2, and 3 are incorrect.
   B. 2 and 3 are correct.
   C. 1, 2, and 3 are correct.

2. Safety should be built into every operation. When you see an unsafe practice you should

   A. Ignore it; it will go away.
   B. Wait until someone gets hurt, fill out an incident report and then correct the problem.
   C. Correct it on the spot.

3. When a chemical is spilled on a worker, you should

   A. Call an ambulance.
   B. Refer to the MSDS sheets for the action to take.
   C. Dry it off right away with a paper towel.

EVALUATING YOUR FACILITY

1. What safety improvements have you made in your facility in the last year?

2. What is the most frequent safety problem? What can be done to reduce the number of incidents?

Chapter Six:
Facilities and Equipment

LEARNING OBJECTIVES

After this chapter you should be able to

- Understand basic facility requirements,
- Relate the benefits of an on-going maintenance program, and
- Name items that should be a part of a routine maintenance check.

Question #10:
A light bulb burns out at home, what do you do?

A. Throw out the lamp.
   Easy but expensive.

B. Sell the house. The light bulb is only a sign of bigger problems.
   A bit extreme and more expensive.

C. Change the light bulb.
   Effective and cheap.

Money spent on a low-cost, on-going maintenance program can be some of the best money a manager ever spends. Maintenance of the facility helps to keep equipment in good working order, troubleshoots more serious problems, promotes safety and sanitation, and maintains the financial investment. A maintenance walk-through can be completed as part of the sanitation walk-through, and any problems can be noted. Problems should then be addressed immediately either in-house or by contacting the appropriate service technicians.

WALLS, CEILINGS, AND FLOORS

Walls should be washed as they become dirty and then periodically to remove dust and any grease film. Ceilings should also be cleaned of any debris. Check ceiling for cracked, chipped, or completely missing tiles and replace them as needed. Floors (the most preferred are grouted quarry tile) should be checked for cleanliness, especially along the baseboards, as well as for cracked, chipped, or missing tiles. Grouting between tiles should also be checked for erosion.

LIGHTING

Minimum lighting requirements are established for the safety of all foodservice facilities and should be maintained. Adequate lighting makes work safe and dirt visible and is a good initial step in pest control—bugs and rodents typically aren't found in well-lighted places. Regularly replacing bulbs and cleaning lighting fixtures (doing so when no foods are in the area) helps maximize lighting performance. For safety purposes all lights should be completely enclosed to prevent breakage into food products. This can be done by enclosing the lights in a frame with a plastic panel embedded in the ceiling (most common) or by enclosing florescent tubes in clear plastic lighting cylinders.

VENTILATION

If you can't stand the heat, check the ventilation. Properly working exhaust systems help to

- Maintain a more consistent room temperature.
- Remove odors from the kitchen.
- Remove excess steam and vapors from the air.
- Reduce dirt accumulation on walls and ceilings.

The size of the ventilation system will vary with the size of the facility, the types of equipment being used, and the volume of steam, heat, and smoke being produced. The system must be in compliance with local laws for both inside requirements and outside venting. The hood filters should be cleaned routinely. NEVER open unscreened windows to help with ventilation—this just welcomes a host of other problems.

PLUMBING

Problems occur when plumbing is not designed with food safety in mind. In designing and maintaining plumbing in a foodservice operation there can be no chance of

- Backflow (water or other liquids with potential for contamination flowing into the drinkable water).
- Cross-connection (a link between unsafe water or chemicals and drinkable water).
- Back siphonage (the pressure of the drinkable water supply is less than that of a contaminated supply, which is sucked into the drinkable water).

To prevent any contamination of the water supply, use the following precautions:

- Create an **air gap** between the downspout for emptying drinkable water and the drain (for example, between a steam kettle and a drain or the three-compartment sink and floor drain.). An air gap is simply free air space. This is the most reliable method. See chapter 4, Figure 4.1.

- Add blackflow prevention devices between all plumbing connections: hook up hoses and spray arms only to sinks that have a prevention device. These devices should be installed by a licensed plumber.
- Check for any overhead water drain lines for leaks or drips and repair immediately.
- Have the facility inspected by a licensed plumber for any deviations and make corrections as needed.

EQUIPMENT

Cleaning and maintenance can add years to the life of a piece of equipment. Follow up quickly on any problems noted. Check refrigerators and freezers for adequate seals and gaskets. Refrigeration and freezer spaces need to be kept clean, and there are products on the market specifically designed to clean in very cold temperatures. Have ovens routinely calibrated for accurate temperatures. Routinely clean dishmachines with a de-limer and check for any necessary curtain replacement. All newly purchased equipment should have the National Sanitation Foundation seal of safety and cleanability (see Fig. 6.1).

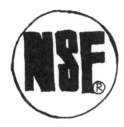

Fig. 6.1. National Sanitation Foundation seal of safety and cleanability.

VENDING MACHINES

All the safety and sanitation precautions for regular foodservice hold true for vended products. Clean trays and slots to remove any sticky buildup that can cause a malfunction. Clean heads, seals, and drip trays of beverage dispensing equipment. Routinely have the machines serviced to maintain appropriate temperatures (perishable foods must remain out of the temperature danger zone). Have water lines for beverage dispensing equipment checked for backflow and buildup.

REST ROOMS, BREAK ROOMS, AND LOCKER ROOMS

These are areas in any facility which are not talked about. But these areas need to be looked at routinely for safety, sanitation, and aesthetic issues. Rest rooms need to be in top functioning order. Plumbing problems need immediate attention. Hand sinks and soap dispensers must be working properly at all times. Hand dryers, single-use paper towels, or continuous-clean cloth rolls must be available for drying; there should be no reusable cloth towels. Break rooms need to have comfortable, sturdy furnishings that are in good repair to promote relaxation. There should be either a cart in the room to hold dirty dishes or another routine established to return items to the kitchen to prevent pest infestation. Locker rooms should be clean and well lit and have adequate storage for personal belongings.

STUDY QUESTIONS

1. The best flooring for a food production area is

   A. Carpet.
   B. Unsealed cement.
   C. Well-grouted quarry tile.

2. Good lighting will

   #1: Improve employee work habits.

   #2: Make soil more visible.

   #3: Reduce the number of pests in the facility.

   A. 1, 2, and 3 are correct.
   B. 1 and 2 are correct.
   C. Only 1 is correct.

3. An effective exhaust system will

   A. Remove stale air, odors, and steam.
   B. Eliminate cleaning of all equipment.
   C. Keep the same air circulating.

4. The most effective backflow-prevention device is

   A. A hose brought in through the back door.
   B. An air gap.
   C. A bucket used to empty the overflow from sinks.

EVALUATING YOUR FACILITY

1. What type of routine is in place at your facility for cleaning and repair of the equipment, walls, ceilings, and floors?

Chapter Seven:
Trash Removal

LEARNING OBJECTIVES

After this chapter you should be able to

■ Identify trash receptacle requirements, and
■ Discuss recycling benefits and needs.

Question #11:
What is trash?

A. Daytime TV?
   Possibly.

B. Most of what you receive in the mail.
   Probably.

C. It means the same thing as the word "politics."
   Definitely.

D. All of the above.
   Yes, and more.

Trash is inevitable. In the daily course of events we are going to create some trash; depending on how things are going, some days we will create much more than others! Trash removal is what the phrase, "it's a dirty job, but somebody's got to do it," refers to. But removing trash properly is another step in the sanitation process.

INDOOR CONTAINERS

According to the FDA Food Code, indoor trash containers must be durable, cleanable, and nonabsorbent. Either there must be a sufficient number of containers to hold trash without overflow or containers must be emptied into an outdoor receptacle prior to overflow. Trash cans should be lined with a heavy, leakproof plastic bag, and they must be covered at all times when not in use. Garbage cans, like all other equipment, must be kept clean. The cleaning process must be done away from food and production areas.

OUTDOOR CONTAINERS

These containers must also be durable, cleanable, and nonabsorbent. They should also be leakproof, and insect and rodent resistant—this means no plastic containers outside.

The container should fit flush to the ground to prevent pest problems underneath. If the container is a dumpster on rollers, it needs to be on a hard surface (cement, asphalt, or gravel). Containers must have a well-fitting lid or cover. The size of an outdoor container must be sufficient to meet the needs of the pickup schedule. Trash may not build up around the outdoor container. Large facilities can benefit from a trash compactor that compresses the trash and allows more trash per container-load pickup. All containers should be routinely cleaned and sanitized to prevent pest problems.

PULPERS

Pulpers are machines that use water to chop waste into small, compact pieces. Although most of the water is removed from the waste after chopping, the result is a dense, moist, heavy waste. Use of pulpers is an effective method of trash compaction, but very-heavy-duty plastic bags must be used to sustain the weight of the final product. The pulper must be cleaned after each use.

RECYCLING

Recycling has now become a routine part of the trash system. Many facilities routinely separate cans, plastics, glass, paper, cardboard, and used cooking oil. Container regulations apply to these items as well: the containers need to be covered, leakproof, and of an adequate number to meet the needs of the facility between pickups. Containers all need to be a part of the routine cleaning schedule. To control odors, flies, and other pests, all recyclables must be thoroughly rinsed of their contents before they are placed in the recycling container. To maximize space, crush cans and plastic before placing them in recyling bins—this is known as volume reduction.

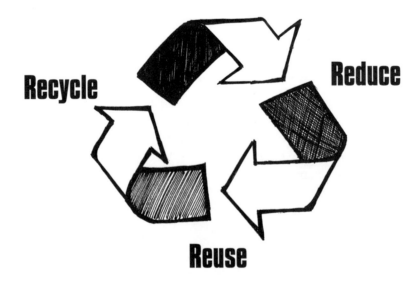

Fig. 7.1. Recycling symbol.

STUDY QUESTIONS

1. All trash containers must be
   A. Cleanable.
   B. Absorbent.
   C. Without a cover.

2. Be a wise owl:
   A. Give a hoot, pollute.
   B. Pile the trash high around the dumpster.
   C. Reduce, reuse, recycle.

EVALUATING YOUR FACILITY

1. What is your biggest source of trash? How can that be reduced?

Chapter Eight

Pest Control

LEARNING OBJECTIVES

After this chapter you should be able to

- Discuss the benefits of an ongoing pest control program and
- Identify the different methods of pest control and their benefits and weaknesses.

Question #12:
The definition of pest control is

A. Keeping your mother-in-law away.
   No comment.

B. Maintaining a file on old boyfriends at the police department.
   No comment.

C. Getting rid of small bugs and rodents that tend to give a large part of the population the willies.
   Kill! Kill!!!

Pest control is essential to food service sanitation: flies, insects, and rodents contaminate food whenever they come into contact with it. A system should be in place for routine checks by an outside pest control company. Pest control companies can develop what is called an Integrated Pest Management (IPM) system which uses a combination of nonchemical and chemical controls to eliminate pests and reduce the use of pesticides. This, in conjunction with a well-used cleaning schedule and timely trash removal, will greatly diminish the opportunity for problems to develop. Pest control should be initiated early because prevention is much more effective than extermination in keeping pests out of buildings.

FLIES

Flies are attracted to garbage and anywhere food is handled. Since they feed off garbage, they are transmitters of several foodborne illnesses. They have no teeth, so they must vomit on solid food, let the food dissolve, and then eat it. To reproduce, flies need moist, decaying materials protected by shade to lay their eggs and have them hatch. Flies reproduce quickly: maggots (hatched eggs) grow into flies in as little as six days.

Control Methods
Remove moist, warm foods, keep trash tightly covered, and close doors after each use. Check door edges and seals and repair any gaps. Clean both indoor and outdoor trash containers regularly. Electric fly traps that electrocute flies can be used around non-food areas but must be designed to retain the bugs within the device. These devices can NOT be located near food production areas. Fans can provide a strong air current at entryways that can prevent flies from entering the kitchen. Nonresidual spray insecticides can be used in food production areas, but label directions MUST be followed.

Residue sprays, which leave a film of insecticide, work well in corners, cracks, and crevices away from food contact areas. Other control methods should be applied by a professional exterminator.

ROACHES

Roaches are another disease-spreading insect. Roaches are partial to warm, dark, hard-to-reach places such as motors, crevices, soft-drink machines, water pipes, and drainage areas. They easily hide under shelves and wallpaper, under rubber matting, and in delivery boxes. They unfortunately can have a life cycle as long as three months to a year. There is often a strong oily odor associated with roaches. Since roaches are partial to darkness, a roach seen in the daylight is a sign of significant infestation.

Control Methods
Check deliveries carefully, refusing anything with signs of bugs. Seal cracks, holes, and crevices. Repair leaks. Keep all foods off the floor and in tightly closed containers. Contact spray, which requires that the spray come in direct contact with the roach, is effective but needs to remain WELL away from any food preparation. Glue traps can be set in warm, dark corners away from food production and storage areas to see if roaches are in the facility, but further treatment should be provided by a pest control specialist.

OTHER BUGS

Weevils, beetles, and moths are typically found in dry storage areas, feeding on grain products and dried beans.

Control Methods
Control methods include checking deliveries for any signs of problems (open bags of flour, for example), keeping foods at least six inches off the floor, rotating stock using FIFO, maintaining a cool temperature in storage areas, and keeping storeroom floors and preparation areas clean.

RODENTS

Rodents carry and spread disease, ruin food, and damage property—they are a serious problem. Rodents can spread germs quickly through urine, feces, and any physical contact with food. Signs of mice and/or rat problems include droppings (new ones are shiny black, old ones are gray), tracks through any dusty surface, holes or dirt piles along foundations, holes in wood or gnawed edges of cardboard, shreds of paper or other materials used to make a nest. Any opening 1/4 inch or larger will let mice in; openings 1/2 inch or larger will allow rats to get in. Rats and mice breed quickly and often create a serious problem in a short amount of time.

Control Methods
Use heavy-duty outdoor trash containers (no plastics—rodents can gnaw through plastic) with tight-fitting lids. Trash containers should be off the ground if possible. Keep all doors and windows shut as much as possible. Glue traps and live traps can help catch rodents, but it is best to get the help of a professional. Poison is to be used ONLY by a licensed professional.

BIRDS

Birds are mostly an exterior problem. They can nest in eaves or overhangs and leave droppings that can make people sick.

Control Methods
Bird control should be left to a pest control company since these companies can use a number of different products to rid the facility of unwanted birds.

For the best possible benefits from an outside pest control company, get what you want in writing. It is best for everyone concerned to spell out exactly what is expected—length of service, number of treatments, materials to be used, and emergency service possibilities. The pest control company should provide Material Safety Data Sheets for all chemicals to be used in the facility. Follow-up should also be outlined so problems can be treated and/or to determine that the facility is currently pest free.

STUDY QUESTIONS

1. In order to keep your facility free of pests, you should have an Integrated Pest Management (IPM) system in place and

    A. A buildup of trash.
    B. An effective cleaning schedule in place.
    C. Mouse traps.

2. What is the best method to detect a pest problem?

    A. An open can of tuna.
    B. Observing your facility in the dark.
    C. A glue board.

EVALUATING YOUR FACILITY

1. What does your facility do for pest management? What improvements could be made?

Chapter Nine:
Inspections

LEARNING OBJECTIVES

After this chapter you should be able to

- Name the benefits of the inspection process,
- List the items health inspectors are most concerned with, and
- Discuss how a HACCP program could improve inspection results.

> *Question #13:*
> *What is worse than Mondays?*
>
> A. Nothing—there is a grassroots movement to lower the number of Mondays from 52 to 15 per year.
> *I'll vote for that.*
>
> B. Mondays and rain.
> *A Carpenters' song?*
>
> C. Being inspected.
> *It doesn't have to be.*

Inspections are synonymous with root canal in terms of fun—nobody wants one. They are, however, necessary and can actually be beneficial. Federal, state, and local laws all play a part in developing the standards for foodservice safety and sanitation requirements. The FDA recommends inspections be every six months, but they are not the primary source of these routine inspections; the FDA's role is to develop food codes and standards for states to use and adapt. State (department of inspection and appeals) and local agencies will be the most directly involved in the inspection process, and they are free to schedule inspections based on workload, prior problems, or an at-risk clientele (elderly or ill). Health care facilities are also frequently involved with federal inspections. Most health inspections are looking for evidence of the following good practices:

- Food is purchased from approved sources in good condition.
- Food storage is prompt and adequate.
- Food production is done appropriately—no cross-contamination.
- Times and temperatures are being observed.
- Equipment is clean and in good working order—there are separate thermometers (not factory installed) placed in the warmest area of all refrigeration units.
- Proper washing and sanitizing of surfaces, pans, and dishware.
- Appropriate hand-washing is being done at an easily accessible sink.

■ Water source is safe and plumbing is appropriate to prevent any backflow.
■ Personal hygiene practices are good.
■ A pest control system is in place.
■ Hazardous chemicals are marked and stored away from food products.

An inspection typically occurs without warning. The inspector should be able to tell you if the inspection is a routine visit, is in response to a complaint, or is for another purpose. Be with the inspector as he/she does a walk-through of the kitchen. Be cooperative, answering any questions or supplying written information. Take notes to write down any comments that you will want to act upon later. Correct as many problems as possible prior to the inspector's leaving the facility. Once the inspection report is completed, study it for problem areas to focus on and discuss the report with staff. Correct any violations within the time frame allowed.

STUDY QUESTIONS

1. How do you get the most out of an inspection?

   A. Be cooperative, correct violations on the spot if possible.
   B. Don't let inspectors in.
   C. Show the inspector your self-check list and tell them you don't need a follow-up report or inspection.

2. Inspections are important to

   A. Be sure food is safe in storage and production.
   B. Explain codes and be sure consumers are safe.
   C. A and B are correct.

EVALUATING YOUR FACILITY

1. What was the score of your last inspection? Have you permanently corrected any noted problems?

Appendixes

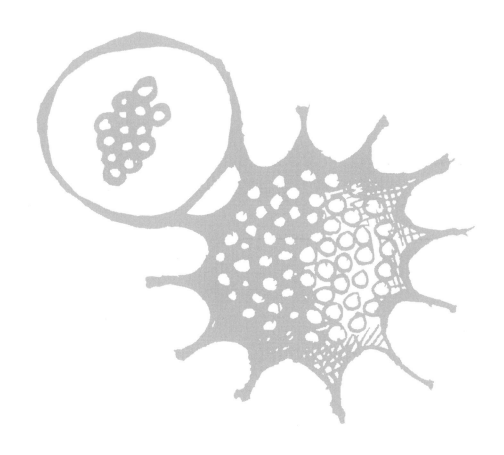

HAZARD ANALYSIS CRITICAL CONTROL POINTS FLOWCHART

Date: _____   Time Started: _____

Product: _____   Time Ended: _____

Main Ingredients: _____   Start - Stop: _____

_____   Less than 4 Hours Total Handling

_____   Time: Yes   No

Recipe Step	Potential Hazard	CCP*	Control/Solution*

Comments: _____

_____

_____

_____

Completed By: _____

ESTABLISHING CORRECTIVE ACTION

CCP	CONTROLS/SOLUTION
Source	Refuse products from unapproved sources.
Delivery	If the product is not in good condition or does not meet specifications, send it back.
Cooking	If the product is not cooked to the proper temperature, pull it from service and reheat above 165°F.
Handling	If cross-contamination occurs, destroy the product.
Holding	If the product is in the danger zone, correct the holding temperature. If the product has been in the danger zone for more than 4 hours, discard it.
Chilling	If the product does not reach 70°F in 2 hours and 40°F in 4 more hours, discard it.
Reheating	If the product has been reheated once, discard the remainder. If it has not been reheated to 165°F, toss it.
Serving	If the product has been handled incorrectly at any of the above control points, DO NOT SERVE IT.

SANITATION WALK-THROUGH

DATE:_____

RECEIVING AREA

ITEM	CLEAN/YES	NEED TO CLEAN/NO	PROBLEM METHOD TO CORRECT	PERSON TO CORRECT
Exterior area				
No trash near entrance				
No openings or holes				
Outside doors				
No signs of bugs/rodents				
Receiving floor clean				
Shelving clean				
Each shipment is checked at the time of delivery for accuracy, spoilage, and any foreign objects (bugs, metal shavings, etc.)				
Refrigerated and frozen products are checked for appropriate temperatures				
Dented cans/pickup items are separated from other product				
Lighting is clean and working				

SANITATION WALK-THROUGH

DATE:_____

SALAD PREP AREA

ITEM	CLEAN/YES	NEED TO CLEAN/NO	PROBLEM METHOD TO CORRECT	PERSON TO CORRECT
Refrigeration				
Separate thermometer in each refrigerator				
Thermometers read below 40°F				
Outsides are clean, including handles				
Insides are clean				
Products are covered, labeled, and dated				
Open products are transferred out of tin cans				
Prep sink is clean				
Work tables are clean and sanitized before and between tasks				
Drawers are clean				
Gloves are worn during cold food preparation				
Shelving is clean				
Utensils are clean and stored properly				
Pans and bowls are clean and stored upside down				
Can openers are clean and free of metal shavings				
Equipment is in working order, clean, and sanitized (check underneath)				
All fresh products are washed before using				
Lighting is adequate and clean				
Floors are clean				
Walls are clean				
Clean sanitizer solution is available in work area				

SANITATION WALK-THROUGH

DATE:_____

COOK/BAKERY PREP AREA

ITEM	CLEAN/YES	NEED TO CLEAN/NO	PROBLEM METHOD TO CORRECT	PERSON TO CORRECT
Refrigeration				
Separate thermometer in each refrigerator				
Thermometers read below 40°F				
Outsides are clean, including handles				
Insides are clean				
Products are covered, labeled, and dated				
Open products are transferred out of tin cans				
All raw meat products are stored on the lowest shelves				
All raw meat products are refrigerated until needed				
All cooked products are heated to appropriate temperatures				
All leftovers are reheated above 165°F				
Work tables are clean and sanitized between tasks				
Drawers are clean				
Shelving is clean				
Utensils are clean and stored properly				
Pans and bowls are clean and stored upside down				
Can openers are clean and free of metal shavings				
Equipment is in working order, clean, and sanitized (check underneath)				
Range hoods are clean and grease free				

SANITATION WALK-THROUGH

DATE:_____

COOK/BAKERY PREP AREA (continued)

ITEM	CLEAN/YES	NEED TO CLEAN/NO	PROBLEM METHOD TO CORRECT	PERSON TO CORRECT
Used grease is properly disposed of				
Sugar and flour bins are clean and scoops are removed				
Spices are in clean containers and covered				
Floors are clean				
Lighting is adequate and clean				
Walls are clean				
Clean sanitizer solution is available in work area				

SANITATION WALK-THROUGH

DATE:_____

TRASH REMOVAL

ITEM	CLEAN/YES	NEED TO CLEAN/NO	PROBLEM METHOD TO CORRECT	PERSON TO CORRECT
All garbage cans are clean, lined, and covered				
Outdoor trash is in a covered container; no trash is on the ground				
Dumpster is in good working condition				
Recyclables are rinsed and placed in appropriate containers				
No signs of bugs/rodents				

SANITATION WALK-THROUGH

DATE:_____

POTS AND PANS

ITEM	CLEAN/YES	NEED TO CLEAN/NO	PROBLEM METHOD TO CORRECT	PERSON TO CORRECT
Scraping, disposal, and power-spray area is in good working order and clean				
All items are scraped or flushed prior to washing				
Wash water is free of grease, and water temperature is appropriate				
Rinse water is clear, and water temperature is appropriate				
Sanitizing solution is checked with a test kit				
Items are air dried on a clean counter				
Floor mats or nonskid surface is in place				
Air gap space is free of any blockage				
Floors are clean and wiped of any large water spills				
Lighting is adequate and clean				
Walls are clean				

SANITATION WALK-THROUGH

DATE:_____

DISHWASHING

ITEM	CLEAN/YES	NEED TO CLEAN/NO	PROBLEM METHOD TO CORRECT	PERSON TO CORRECT
Dishes are scraped before racking				
Racks are uncrowded				
Dishmachine compartments are at the appropriate temperatures				
Adequate chemical supply is available				
Silverware is run through the machine twice				
Dishes are air dried before being put away				
Dishes are stored on dish carts or lowerators or stacked face down on matted shelving				
All dish storage equipment is clean and sanitized				
Floor mats or nonskid surface is in place				
Air-gap space is free of any blockage				
Dishmachine is free of lime buildup				
Floors are clean and wiped of any large water spills				
Lighting is adequate and clean				
Walls are clean				

SANITATION WALK-THROUGH

DATE:_____

DRY STORAGE

ITEM	CLEAN/YES	NEED TO CLEAN/NO	PROBLEM METHOD TO CORRECT	PERSON TO CORRECT
Adequate shelving to store all products				
Bottom shelves are at least 6" off the ground				
FIFO method is being used with products				
Opened products are stored in covered, labeled, and dated containers				
Chemical storage is separated from food storage				
All foods and chemicals have readable labels				
All dented cans have been removed				
No signs of bugs/rodents				
Temperature is between 60° and 70°F				
Shelving and cans are free of dust and dirt				
Nothing is stored under wastewater pipes				
Lighting is adequate and clean				
Walls are clean				

SANITATION WALK-THROUGH

DATE:_____

COLD STORAGE

ITEM	CLEAN/YES	NEED TO CLEAN/NO	PROBLEM METHOD TO CORRECT	PERSON TO CORRECT
Walk-in temperature is below 40°F on a separate thermometer				
Freezer temperature is below 0°F on a separate thermometer				
Shelving is clean				
No trays or papers on shelving				
Doors close properly; seals are in good condition				
All foods are at least 6" off the floor				
All foods are covered, labeled, and dated				
Cooked products are stored in containers less than 4" deep to cool				
Frozen foods are thawed under refrigeration				
FIFO method is being used with all products				
Fan and coils are dust free				
Freezers are defrosted as needed				
Lighting is adequate and clean				
Floors are clean				
Walls are clean				

SANITATION WALK-THROUGH

DATE:_____

SERVING AREA

ITEM	CLEAN/YES	NEED TO CLEAN/NO	PROBLEM METHOD TO CORRECT	PERSON TO CORRECT
Serving area is protected from customers by a clean Plexiglas guard				
Items are being held at the proper temperatures: Hot foods above 140°F Cold foods below 40°F				
Every item has its own serving utensil stored in the product				
Gloves are worn when handling cold or raw food products				
Salad bars are protected by a clean sneeze guard				
Return trips to a salad bar are done with a clean dish				
Glassware is stored with the drinking rim down				
Silverware is stored with the eating ends down				
Lighting is adequate and clean				
Floor is clean				
Walls are clean				

SANITATION WALK-THROUGH

DATE:_____

EMPLOYEES

ITEM	CLEAN/YES	NEED TO CLEAN/NO	PROBLEM METHOD TO CORRECT	PERSON TO CORRECT
Uniforms and aprons are clean				
Hair is restrained appropri- ately				
Closed-toe, leather, nonskid shoes are worn				
Handwashing is done at the beginning of the shift and after each break from work				
Cuts are covered with a bandage and a disposable glove				
Disposable gloves are changed frequently				
Disposable gloves are used to handle and serve foods that are served uncooked				
Thermometers are available and are used to test temperatures				
Jewelry is limited				
Fingernails are clean and short; no false nails are worn				
No smoking or gum chewing in work area				
No beverages in work area				

SANITATION WALK-THROUGH

DATE:_____

BEVERAGES

ITEM	CLEAN/YES	NEED TO CLEAN/NO	PROBLEM METHOD TO CORRECT	PERSON TO CORRECT
Coffee urns are clean and free of residue				
Ice machines are in good working order and clean				
Nothing but ice scoops are used to get ice out				
Ice scoops are not left in the machine				
Juice-, pop-, and milk-dispensing equipment is clean				
Dispensing heads are sanitized daily				
Refrigerated dispensers are maintained below 40°F				

SANITATION WALK-THROUGH

DATE:_____

GENERAL

ITEM	CLEAN/YES	NEED TO CLEAN/NO	PROBLEM METHOD TO CORRECT	PERSON TO CORRECT
Hand sinks are in good working condition, cleaned, and stocked				
Rolling carts are clean and sturdy				
Vending machines and vending area are clean				
Proper temperatures are maintained in vending equipment				
Restrooms are clean				
Restrooms have adequate soap and paper supplies				

Completed By: _____

MAXIMUM RECOMMENDED STORAGE TIMES (REFRIGERATOR/FREEZER)

FOOD ITEM	TIME IN REFRIGERATOR AT 35°–40°F	TIME IN FREEZER AT 0°F
Meats		
Ground, stew meat	1 to 2 days	3 to 4 months
Variety meats	1 to 2 days	3 to 4 months
Chops, ribs	2 to 3 days	3 to 6 months
Steaks	3 to 5 days	6 to 12 months
Roasts	3 to 5 days	6 to 12 months
Cooked meats, leftover	1 to 2 days	2 to 3 months
Cured and smoked meats		
Bacon	5 to 7 days	1 month
Corned beef	5 to 7 days	2 weeks
Ham, canned	6 months	Not recommended
Ham, sliced	3 to 4 days	Not recommended
Ham, picnic	5 to 7 days	Not recommended (Due to flavor and texture changes)
Sausage	2 to 3 weeks	Not recommended
Hot dogs	4 to 5 days	1 month
Luncheon meats	1 week	Not recommended
Smoked sausage	1 week	Not recommended
Poultry		
Chicken, duck, turkey	1 to 2 days	6 to 7 months
Cooked poultry	1 day	2 to 3 months
Giblets	1 day	3 months
Fish		
Fresh, fatty (salmon)	1 to 2 days	3 months
Fresh	2 to 3 days—iced	6 months
Shellfish	1 to 2 days	3 to 4 months
Eggs		
Raw in shell	3 weeks	Not recommended
Leftover cracked eggs	2 days	Not recommended
Reconstituted eggs	1 week	Not recommended
Liquid eggs, open	3 days	Do not refreeze
Liquid eggs, unopened	10 days	Do not refreeze
Dairy		
Milk	5 to 7 days after carton date	Not recommended
Butter	2 weeks	3 to 6 months
Hard cheese (cheddar)	5 to 6 months	Not recommended
Soft cheeses (cream, brie)	3 days	Not recommended
Cottage cheese	1 week	Not recommended
Reconstituted milk	1 week	Not recommended
Ice cream	NA	3 months
Mayonnaise, opened	2 months	Not recommended

MAXIMUM RECOMMENDED STORAGE TIMES (STOREROOM)

FOOD ITEM	TIME IN STOREROOM AT 70°F
Baking supplies	
Baking powder/soda	8 to 12 months
Baking chocolate	8 to 12 months
Cornstarch	2 to 3 years
Flour	9 to 12 months
Sugar	Indefinite
Tapioca	1 year
Dry yeast	1 to 1 1/2 years
Canned items	
Condensed or evaporated milk	1 year
Fruits and vegetables	1 to 2 years
Fruit juices	6 to 9 months
Soups	1 year
Tuna, salmon, etc.	1 year
Coffee	
Not vacuum packed	2 weeks
Vacuum packed	8 to 12 months
Instant	8 to 12 months
Condiments	
Mayonnaise	6 months
Mustard	2 to 6 months
Oil	6 to 9 months
Pickles	1 year
Relish	1 year
Salad dressings	2 months
Sauces (soy, Worcestershire)	2 years
Shortenings	2 to 4 months
Syrups	1 year
Grains	
Cereals, hot and cold	6 to 8 months
Pasta	3 months
Rice, parboiled	9 to 12 months, refrigerate brown and wild rice
Seasonings	
Herbs	1 to 2 years
Salt	Indefinite
Spices, ground	2 years
Spices, whole	3 to 5 years

Study Question
Answers

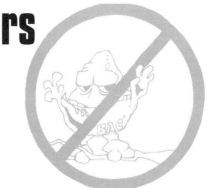

Chapter 1. Food Hazards

1. C—Biological hazards can have the most serious health risks.
2. D
3. B—Heat items to their appropriate temperature and then hold above 140°F.
4. A—The others are also good foodservice practices but won't necessarily affect bacterial growth.

Chapter 2. Foodborne Illnesses

1. C
2. C
3. C
4. A
5. B—The others are good safety precautions but won't control the transmission.
6. A

Chapter 3. Preparation and Service of Safe Food

1. A
2. C
3. C—The others are good control points, but the most likely time for food to be in the temperature danger zone is during preparation and holding.
4. C
5. B
6. A—Because the temperature of the product may not be high enough to kill bacteria. The other two products are heated to at least 145°F.
7. A
8. A
9. C
10. C
11. B—#3 is *technically* not cross-contamination because the onion was cut first, and also because both the onion and the turkey will be cooked together to the proper temperature to prevent bacterial growth. But it is BETTER to always use the rule of never mixing raw products (i.e., meat and vegetables) on the same cutting board.

12. D
13. C—A candy thermometer has the wrong temperature range, and glass thermometers have the potential to break.
14. B
15. C
16. C

Chapter 4. Cleaning and Sanitization

1. C
2. C
3. B
4. B

Chapter 5. Safety

1. A
2. C
3. B

Chapter 6. Facilities and Equipment

1. C
2. A—Pests don't like well-lit places.
3. A
4. B

Chapter 7. Trash Removal

1. A
2. C

Chapter 8. Pest Control

1. B
2. C—A glue board will give you indications of further infestation.

Chapter 9. Inspections

1. A
2. C

Glossary

ACIDIC

having acid quality. A low pH level—the more acidic (below 4.5), the less likely bacterial growth will occur.

AIRFLOW

is the ability for air to freely circulate. The better the airflow the easier it is to cool products down and maintain temperatures.

AIR GAP

the free space between the lowest piece of pipe from a water supply and the drain.

ASEPTIC

free of infection. Prevention of contact with microorganisms. A method of packaging that prevents contamination from microorganisms, prolonging shelf life.

BACKFLOW

the reverse flow of dirty water into the clean water due to greater pressure.

BACTERIA

any of a large group of microscopic plants, including some that are disease producers.

CARRIER

one that transports an infectious agent while remaining well him- or herself.

CHELATION

the use of an organic compound to attach to water-hardness particles. This allows for better cleaning and sanitizing of dishware.

CLEAN

free of dirt or waste by the use of hot water and appropriate detergent.

CONTACT SPRAY

an insecticide that makes actual contact with the bug. This must be done away from food preparation areas.

CONTAMINATION

infection by contact with undesirable organisms.

CRITICAL CONTROL POINT

a spot along the food preparation path that can have to a direct effect on the safe outcome of a food product (i.e., thawing meat). Once these points are identified, systems can be put in place to check that proper practices are being followed.

CROSS-CONNECTION

a pipe connection that potentially allows for unsafe water to flow into the clean water supply. This would need immediate attention to correct.

CROSS-CONTAMINATION

transfer of harmful organisms from one food to another by way of a food contact surface (i.e., cutting board, counter top, knife, hands, etc.).

DANGER ZONE

temperatures at which bacteria grow best—40° to 140°F. Foods need to be passed quickly through this temperature zone by rapid cooling or heating.

DE-LIMER

a chemical agent to remove lime deposits, primarily in dish machines.

ENDOTOXIN

a toxin produced in a microorganism and released when the microorganism disintegrates.

FIFO

first in, first out method of product rotation. By using the products that came into the facility first there is less chance of spoilage.

FOODBORNE ILLNESS

disease or illness obtained through the consumption of contaminated food.

FOOD CONTACT SURFACE

a surface that has the potential to come into direct contact with food or items used for food preparation.

FUNGI

organisms without chlorophyll or a rigid cell wall—including mushrooms, yeasts, and molds.

GLUE TRAPS

a contained pest control method with a sticky, poisonous substance along the bottom when placed on the floor that the pest will walk across and get stuck.

HACCP

Hazard Analysis Critical Control Points—a system of checks to maintain the safest food possible from purchasing through service.

HAZARDS

are items that when in contact with foods can pose a safety threat. They are divided into three categories: Physical hazards—any object (hair, dirt, metal shavings, etc.) that can fall onto food products; Chemical hazards—any exposure to the absorption of chemicals (cleaners, pest control products, etc.); Biological hazards—organisms that grow in or are transported to foods to produce a foodborne illness.

HOST

an animal or plant on which a parasite lives.

IMMERSION

to plunge deep into a liquid, to be completely covered.

INSECTICIDE

any chemical substance which kills insects.

INTEGRATED PEST MANAGEMENT (IPM)

IPM—a complete pest control program that looks at ways to eliminate present pest problems as well as future prevention measures. This usually includes the services of an outside pest management company.

MATERIAL SAFETY DATA SHEET (MSDS)

MSDS—a safety sheet required for all hazardous compounds in a facility. Each sheet provides information about the product, its uses, precautions, and how to handle physical contact problems.

MICROORGANISM

a living being only seen by a microscope.

MODIFIED ATMOSPHERE PACKAGING (MAP)

MAP—a sealed package that has replaced oxygen with other gases to improve the product's shelf life.

Nonresidual pesticide

a pesticide that works quickly and then becomes ineffective in several hours.

Outbreak

two or more people experiencing the same illness after eating the same food product(s) as confirmed through laboratory analysis. In cases of botulism, due to the severity of the problems, one person's illness is considered an outbreak.

Parasite

a plant or animal living on another organism at the host's expense.

Pasteurization

heating foods to a temperature that destroys harmful bacteria.

Pathogenic

those microorganisms that are disease producing.

pH

the negative logarithm of the effective hydrogen concentration. A way to express acidity and alkalinity. pHs of 4.6 to 7.0 are considered optimal for bacteria to grow.

Potentially hazardous foods

are those foods that are high in moisture and protein, giving bacteria the optimal growing conditions.

Repellent

a substance used to prevent insect attacks, which does not necessarily kill the insects.

Residual spray

is a film of insecticide used mostly in cracks and creases to kill insects that crawl across it. Cannot be used near food contact surfaces.

Sanitize

reduce or eliminate bacteria to levels that will not cause foodborne illness.

Spore

an inactive bacterial cell that can withstand extreme hot and cold fluctuations. Spores can germinate, becoming capable of reproduction.

SURFACTANT

a surface active agent—soaps and detergents—that ease the surface tension to allow dirt to be removed.

TOXIN

substance produced by living organisms that is very poisonous.

UHT PACKAGING

ultra-pasteurized, aseptically packaged food products. This is done by high temperatures for short time periods. Provides longer shelf life and does not need refrigeration until after the package is opened.

VEGETATIVE CELL

an active bacteria, able to reproduce. Can be killed by high temperatures.

VENTILATION

circulation of air, the process of providing fresh air. The process removes heat, smoke, and steam from the area.

VIRUS

a tiny infective agent, it is protein-wrapped genetic material, which is only able to replicate within a living host cell.

WATER HARDNESS

water with a high supply of magnesium and calcium.

WHOLESOME

food that is clean, free of contamination, and safe to eat.

References

American Egg Board, *The Egg Handling and Care Guide*, Park Ridge, IL, September 1994.

Ecolab, Inc., Institutional Division.

FDA, Center for Food Safety and Applied Nutrition, *Foodborne Pathogenic Microorganisms and Natural Toxins Handbook*, 1997.

FDA, Office of Seafood.

FDA, Public Health Service, Department of Health and Human Services, 1997 Food Code.

FDA, *Can Your Kitchen Pass the Food Safety Test?* FDA Consumer, November 1996, Publication No. (FDA) 98-1229.

Food Service Establishment Laws and Rules, Iowa Department of Inspections and Appeals, Des Moines, IA, 1997.

Food Service Establishment Laws and Rules, Iowa Department of Inspections and Appeals 1999 Updates, Des Moines, IA.

Illinois State Health Codes, 1996.

International Food Information Council, *Food Insight: Current Topics in Food Safety and Nutrition*, July 1998.

Iowa State University Extension, *Food Safety Project*, 1997.

McDermott, Karen G., "Putting HACCP to Work," *Restaurants and Institutions, 1997*, p. 34.

National Cattlemen's Beef Association, *Foodservice Ground Beef Safety*, Chicago, IL, 1996.

National Center for Infectious Diseases, Center for Disease Control and Prevention, Division of Bacterial and Mycotic Diseases, *Preventing Foodborne Illness*, Atlanta, GA, August 1996.

National Center for Infectious Diseases, Center for Disease Control and Prevention, Food and Water Borne Bacterial Diseases, Atlanta, GA, 1997.

National Frozen Food Association, *Safety First—Taking Temperature*, A supplement to Restaurant Business, Inc., Publications, 1998.

National Pork Producers, *Food Safety*, Des Moines, IA, 1998.

NSF International, *Recommended Field Procedures for Spray-type Dishwashing Machines*, 1982.

Tone's Spices, Des Moines, IA.

University of California Cooperative Extension, *Ensuring Food Safety the HACCP Way*, Davis, CA, 1998.

USDA, Food Safety and Inspection Service, *The Seven HACCP Principles*, February 1998.

USDA, Meat and Poultry Hotline, *Food Safety Features*, September 1997.

USDA, Economic Research Service, *Foodborne Illness Costs from Seven Major Pathogens*, August 1996.

Washington State University Cooperative Extension, *Foodborne Botulism*, Spokane, WA, 1998.